LARYNGECTOMEE SPEECH
AND
REHABILITATION

LARYNGECTOMEE SPEECH AND REHABILITATION

By

WARREN H. GARDNER, Ph.D., F.A.S.H.A.

*Founder, International Association
of Laryngectomees*

Formerly

*Professor, Hearing and Speech Therapy
Western Reserve University*

*Director of Clinical Services
Cleveland Hearing and Speech Center*

*Chief, Speech Pathology and Audiology
Department of Otolaryngology
Cleveland Clinic Foundation*

President, American Hearing Society

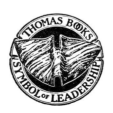

CHARLES C THOMAS • PUBLISHER
Springfield • Illinois • U.S.A.

Published and Distributed Throughout the World by

CHARLES C THOMAS • PUBLISHER

BANNERSTONE HOUSE

301–327 East Lawrence Avenue, Springfield, Illinois, U.S.A.

NATCHEZ PLANTATION HOUSE

735 North Atlantic Boulevard, Fort Lauderdale, Florida, U.S.A.

© *1971, by* CHARLES C THOMAS • PUBLISHER

Library of Congress Catalog Card Number: 72–130927

With THOMAS BOOKS *careful attention is given to all details of*
manufacturing and design. It is the Publisher's desire to present books
that are satisfactory as to their physical qualities and artistic possibilities
and appropriate for their particular use. THOMAS BOOKS *will be true*
to those laws of quality that assure a good name and good will.

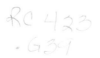

Printed in the United States of America

BB-14

To my wife, Dorothy,

who patiently endured my absence
while I researched and wrote this book

PREFACE

This book was written for the purpose of giving a practical, clinical orientation to the teacher of esophageal speech and of speech with the artificial larynx. It has been designed to acquaint the reader with a program of rehabilitation that begins with the patient's first interview with the surgeon and terminates with (hopefully) adequate communication, return to work and renewed friendships.

The author has witnessed in over a quarter of a century, the appearance of a relatively new type of speech disorder and a new name for a patient who has this speech defect. Modern medicine, surgery and nursing techniques have enabled laryngectomees to survive. The rapid increase in their numbers and the dramatic change in their speech has stimulated speech pathologists and laryngologists to study their problems. The outpouring of research findings in the last twenty years has shown us how greatly the new voice differs from the natural voice, and how seriously the loss of voice affects the lives of laryngectomized persons.

The author has endeavored to give the reader the minimal amount of medical information that will still enable him to understand the background of the laryngectomized patient. He has emphasized throughout the text the clinical aspects of rehabilitation, that is, how best to help the teacher of esophageal speech to solve the complex problems associated with loss of speech through laryngectomy. He has given ample references for those who wish to delve more deeply into some particular aspect of this new area of speech pathology.

The university professor may use this book as a basic plan of rehabilitation to which he can add and subtract information and treatment procedures which he has found to be successful. The book may also be used by the laryngectomee both to understand the psychophysiological aspects of his own speech problem and for self-instruction.

Many persons, knowingly or unknowingly, have contributed to the many bits and pieces of this book. I wish to express my deep appreciation to Charles Van Riper, Ph.D., author of many speech textbooks, for his encouragement to complete this book. I thank William M. Diedrich, Ph.D., and James Shanks, Ph.D., for their patient and thoughtful evaluation of the manuscript and their suggestions that improved the clarity and authenticity of the material; Willard Parker, M.D., who made helpful suggestions on the surgical aspects of laryngectomy, and V. F. Pekarek, M.D., a laryngectomized surgeon and advisor to the Cleveland Lost Chord Club, who supplied information on hygiene of the stoma, first aid and safety, and whose conversations through the years have stimulated many ideas for giving better service to the laryngectomee through Lost Chord Club activities.

I am deeply appreciative of the early work with laryngectomees in Cleveland by Julius McCall, M.D., who, with Amy Bishop Foster, founded the Cleveland Lost Chord Club in 1947 at the Cleveland Hearing and Speech Center, and who remained the club's adviser for many years. I also wish to give thanks to Harold E. Harris, M.D.; Fred R. Tingwald, M.D., and Willard Parker, M.D., of the Cleveland Clinic Foundation for their interest and cooperation in developing the patient orientation and instruction program for laryngectomees in a hospital-clinic setup.

I am very grateful for the privilege of meeting and working with the many laryngectomees of the Cleveland Lost Chord Club and with those who sought consultation at the nineteen conventions of the International Association of Laryngectomees. I have an especially fond memory of the members of the Speech Standards Committee of the IAL, who conducted the many speech programs at the conventions and who contributed substantially to the improvement of standards for teaching esophageal speech.

I must not forget the generous contribution of the Cuyahoga Unit of the American Cancer Society, in Cleveland, Ohio, through Mrs. Patricia Palmer, Director. That contribution and the financial support of the National Cancer Institute of the National Institutes of Health enabled me, aided by the business management of George J. Fortune, Director of the Cleveland Hearing and Speech Center, to found the IAL in 1952. The succeeding financial sponsor, the American Cancer Society, and its excellent staff, likewise should be commended for carrying the financial burden of the IAL from its early days, and for counseling the directors of the young association, which has since become internationally known. The IAL began with ten chartered clubs; there are now 145 clubs in ten nations, as well as many nonaffiliated groups. In addition to the contribution mentioned above, the Cuyahoga Unit of the American Cancer Society has continued to finance the teaching of esophageal speech through grants to the Cleveland Hearing and Speech Center, which in turn has offered its space and services to the club for the past twenty-five years. Finally, I express great appreciation for the wise advice of Charles Taylor of the American Cancer Society and for the great leadership of IAL's executive secretary, Jack Ranney.

I wish to thank the American Medical Association for permission to use photographs which appeared in pages 778, 782, 785 and 786 of the *Archives of Environmental Health,* vol. 9, December 1964, and on pages

147–50 of the *Archives of Otolaryngology*, vol. 73, February 1961. We have acknowledged by appropriate references in the manuscript the quotations, statements and sources of material that substantially enhanced proof of certain important arguments.

I wish to conclude with the admission that many of the explanations within this book could not have been offered if they had not been clarified by my former student Dr. William M. Diedrich, who brought into flower through cinefluorography the reality and understanding of the inner workings (hitherto invisible) of injection and expulsion of air during esophageal speech. He made possible the viewing of the complete sequential action and the simultaneity of action of the different parts of the speech mechanism. Hence, no apologies are offered for the frequent references to Diedrich and Youngstrom's work, as well as to those of Snidecor, Damsté and other contemporary writers, which made this book possible.

INTRODUCTION

Speech pathologists have witnessed within the last thirty years a marked expansion in the rehabilitation of laryngectomized persons. This rehabilitation has largely taken the form of reestablishing the patient's ability to communicate. Communication without the use of the larynx has been known since 1828, when a person with complete atresia of the glottis was able to talk by injecting air into the esophagus (Luchsinger and Arnold). Czermak in 1859 reported that a girl who had total occlusion of the larynx later spontaneously developed an esophageal voice. Another type of alaryngeal communication appeared in 1874 when Billroth's laryngectomized patient survived surgery and was fitted with an artificial larynx (Gussenbauer) The term *pseudovoice* was mentioned by Landois in 1888 (Luchsinger and Arnold, p. 288). Frankel in 1893 located the source of esophageal voice production at the opening of the esophagus into the hypopharynx. Seeman first used the term *esophageal speech* in 1919 (Damsté). The lexicographer of the *Literary Digest* suggested in 1934 that the term *laryngectomee* was a logical name for a laryngectomized person (Ehrlich).

Although laryngectomees generally communicated by instruments in the nineteenth century, an occasional person was able spontaneously to talk with what was thought to be esophageal voice. Communication by esophageal voice became more frequent as improvements in surgery permitted patients to survive In 1908 Gutzmann astonished the medical world by reporting that he had successfully taught twenty-five laryngectomees to talk with esophageal speech.

The mortality rate from cancer of the larynx decreased from 80 per cent prior to 1911 to 10 per cent by 1928 as a result of Mackenty's improvement of surgery from two stages (tracheotomy and a later laryngectomy) to one (McCall 1953). Continued improvements in surgical techniques for shaping the incision and sewing the tracheal stoma to the skin, as well as improvements in nursing techniques, reduced the mortality rate well below 10 per cent (McCall 1953). Finally, the development and use of antibiotics in the late 1930's made it possible for many laryngectomized patients not only to survive the operation but to communicate by esophageal speech or by use of the artificial larynx, and to return to work (Gardner).

The increase in numbers of living laryngectomees has come from two sources. The first which has already been discussed, is the increasing survival rate as a result of improvements in surgery and medicine. The other factor stems from the marked increase of cancer of the throat in recent years. The American Cancer Society has reported that 3,000 laryngectomees yearly survive surgery for cancer of the larynx. The present estimate is that over 23,000 laryngectomees are living in the United States (Snidecor 1968). The increasing numbers of patients have made increasing demands upon surgeons and speech pathologists to restore communication to these people.

The dramatic deprivation of the larynx with all of the complications of physical, physiological, psychological, social and economic problems demands a much broader therapeutic program than has been required of persons who have simpler types of voice defects. Much of the therapeutic program for laryngectomees in the United States has been stimulated by the increased interest of surgeons and speech pathologists in the development of instruction in esophageal speech, and by the publicity programs of the International Association of Laryngectomees and the American Cancer Society. The nineteen annual meetings of the IAL, which have been sponsored by the American Cancer Society, have advertised vividly the need for rehabilitation services for laryngectomees. Indeed, this is one of the important goals of the American Cancer Society. The IAL's institutes for teaching esophageal speech, financially supported by the Office of Vocational Rehabilitation and the American Cancer Society, have trained several hundred laryngectomized teachers and speech pathologists in rehabilitation and in methods of teaching esophageal speech to laryngectomees. University seminars in all parts of the nation also have produced many instructors in esophageal speech. Publications on cancer and surgery of the larynx, and research in alaryngeal morphology, psychophysiology and the communicative aspects of the problems of laryngectomized persons have appeared throughout the world in greatly increasing numbers during the last two decades.*

---

* Read the history of the IAL and an analysis of publications over the past 100 years in Gardner 1962b.

CONTENTS

UNITS OF INSTRUCTION

ESOPHAGEAL SPEECH

LARYNGECTOMEE SPEECH
AND
REHABILITATION

Chapter One

PRELARYNGECTOMY ORIENTATION
OF THE PATIENT

In the early days when cancer of the larynx meant death (McCall 1953), and during the later periods of low survival rate, surgeons were largely concerned with postoperative recovery (Snidecor). They had only a "passive or laissez-faire" attitude toward rehabilitation (Martin 1963). In the present period in which large numbers of victims of cancer of the larynx survive, there is a great need for guiding the patients to solve their communication, physical, emotional, social and economic problems.

Rehabilitation of a laryngectomized person begins during the interview in which the surgeon informs the patient that he has cancer, and that the larynx must be removed (Damsté 1958; Diedrich and Youngstrom; Fontaine and Mitchell; Gardner; Hodson and Oswald; Holinger *et al.*; Kusske; Levin; Luchsinger and Arnold; McCall; Snidecor; Waldrop 1965). The surgeon must be prepared for marked reactions of the patient to this fearful news: cancer, fear of death, loss of speech, loss of job and of friends (Nahum and Golden; Pitkin). Reports in the medical literature indicate that some patients are so disturbed that they attempt or think of suicide (Damsté; Gardner 1966; Heaver *et al.*; Luchsinger and Arnold; Martin; Schall). In Gardner's report many patients were frightened to speechlessness and wept. Others exclaimed, "Why did this happen to me? This is the end." Diedrich and Youngstrom's patients gave similar remarks: "I felt like I was joining the living dead. I will be useless and dependent." However, others calmly accepted the verdict or said, "Glad someone found out what was wrong with me."*

The patient's statement in the last sentence points to the philosophy of this book. We intend to demonstrate that a speech therapy and rehabilitative program will show the patient the way to readjustment of problems associated with loss of voice. We also hope to show that mutual cooperation of the patient and professional people will ease the otherwise distressful problems the patient endures.

The laryngectomee receives three blows to his equanimity when he becomes a victim of cancer of the larynx. The first blow is the news that

---

* Readers may find many items indicative of preoperative unhappiness by reading Diedrich and Youngstrom; Gardner 1966; Horn; Pitkin; and Schall.

3

he has cancer. The second blow is his mental and physical impressions during the immediate postoperative days. Long, a surgeon, wrote of his impressions following his own laryngectomy: "Within a few hours, one loses all real ability to communicate except in writing. A sense of frustration rapidly builds up to devastating proportions." The third blow takes place when the patient appears before the public as a laryngectomee: a man with a hole in his neck. He experiences embarrassment, frustration, a feeling of inferiority and a sense of social and economic failure (Damsté; Gardner 1966; J. S. Greene; Haase; Klieger; Nahum and Golden; Pitkin; Schall 1938, 1954; Stoll).

Since these traumatic episodes occur in a sequence of time, their treatment calls for three stages of adjustment:

1. Preoperative orientation.
2. Immediate postoperative orientation.
3. Restoration and return of the laryngectomee to his original milieu.

These three stages emphasize the importance of continuing guidance not only through the immediate postoperative period, but also throughout the several years in which the laryngectomee strives to rise above personal and physical insults in order to regain his preoperative social and economic status. Since five-year survival is regarded as a cure of this particular type of cancer, the surgeon is an important adviser and counselor for the patient throughout this period.

RESPONSIBILITY OF THE SURGEON

The first and last responsibility for the rehabilitation of the laryngectomee lies in the hands of the surgeon (Gilmore; Haase; Heaver *et al.*; McCall *et al.*; Moses 1965; Nahum and Golden; Pitkin; Schall; Snidecor; Van Riper and Irwin). Moses points out the responsibility of the surgeon when he argues: ". . . he who has taken away the voice is logically the responsible person for restoring this function."* Montreuil states:

> A patient who is about to have his larynx removed thereby loses his voice organ, and requires proper psychological guidance. He must be conditioned in advance and assured that he can be rehabilitated and taught to communicate with his fellow men by means of the esophageal voice.

Martin (1963) protests:

> Since loss of the power of speech is the basic and the outstanding disability in total laryngectomy, it might seem reasonable at first thought that remedial

---

* For a comprehensive outline of the surgeon's duties, see Martin 1963 and Snidecor 1968.

measures be limited simply to the restoration of this function in the restricted form of *esophageal speech* rather than in the broader image of *postlaryngectomy rehabilitation* of speech by the most practical method. In my opinion, the prevalence of such a narrow concept is largely responsible for the shortcomings of present-day services for rehabilitation of the laryngectomee.

The Patient's Anxieties

When the patient is informed by the surgeon that he has cancer of the larynx, a kaleidoscopic train of thoughts about his fate and that of his family rushes through his mind. "Will I live? Will I talk again? Will I get my job back? What will happen to my wife and children? How will my friends react?" While the surgeon is explaining the necessary surgery, the patient's thoughts come so forcefully and rapidly after each other that he cannot absorb or grasp much of what the surgeon tells him. This may explain why some patients complain indignantly that the surgeon did not tell them that the stoma could not be sewn shut (Martin 1955). This situation probably is similar to the experiences of twenty-three of Diedrich and Youngstrom's patients who asserted that they were not told they would no longer be able to breathe through their noses. A good example of one patient's confusion was his answer to a question about what the surgeon had told him: "No plans that I heard—so many things to do."

The Patient's Need for Understanding His Problem

At a time when the patient is still able to talk, to express his feelings and to ask questions, it is very important for the surgeon to take time patiently to explain in a sympathetic and understanding manner that many of the patient's fears are not justified (Nahum and Golden). Removing the cancer may save and prolong his life. The patient will be back with his spouse and children as before. The surgeon should assure the patient that he can begin speech lessons as soon as his wounds are well healed (Levin; Martin 1963). Waldrop and Baker suggest that the surgeon emphasize that the patient will have only a temporary loss of speech. This gives him the belief that he will talk again. The surgeon can also prepare the patient for certain physical changes that he will experience, including the fact that he will breathe through an opening in his throat instead of through his nose. He can assure the patient that he will breathe more easily than persons with a larynx (Pekarek). Kusske states:

> The reason for the type of selected surgery should be understood. That is where a total laryngectomy is indicated. It is well to point out to the patient that his larynx is really useless because of its destruction by cancerous cells.

That in truth, he is not losing anything because it is already destroyed. In a sense, you might point out he's really gaining, by having removed from his body the growth which is endangering his very existence. Thus, giving the patient an insight into his problem, we as doctors will have done much to relieve and to lessen anxieties and tension. The patient should be told that although he's losing his larynx, he will learn to talk again. He is advised that a qualified member of an esophageal speech clinic will see him before surgery. Thus the patient can see for himself that clear and audible speech of good quality can be his with proper training.

The patient will lose the senses of taste and smell at first (Diedrich and Youngstrom; M.C.L. Greene; Horn; Johnson; Kindler; Lindsay *et al.*; Luchsinger and Arnold; Nelson). However, he may regain them to some extent. He will have difficulty in swallowing which will be quickly overcome as it becomes once again a reflex habit. The patient likewise should return to most of the social and sporting activities he enjoyed before, except that he will not be able to swim (Martin 1963; Moses; Schall 1954); some people even do that.*

It is also urgent for the surgeon to warn the patient that he will have marked emotions of regret, frustration and anger (Moses; Schall 1954). He may tell the patient: "You may even be mad at me because I took away your voice but you will soon begin to feel better and be glad that the cancer is out. You must be aware of these feelings and understand that it is natural for anyone who has had part of his body removed to act this way" (Gardner 1954; Morrison; Pitkin). Snidecor suggested that the following preparatory statement about postlaryngectomy speech might be given to the patient:

"I want to warn you, however, it will be no easy job. It probably will be the most frustrating and aggravating task you ever faced and it will take a long time to master it."

One of Diedrich and Youngstrom's patients said that he would give a more radically frank warning if he were asked to visit a prospective laryngectomee:

"Grit your teeth and prepare for an experience more horrible, more terrible, more torturing than you have or could possibly imagine before you experience it. . . ." (Diedrich and Youngstrom)

Some patients probably can withstand such bluntness but we do not believe any surgeon would be so brutally frank or allow any visitant to

* A Belgian laryngectomee swims under water by wearing a tight-fitting tube in his stoma. The other end of the tube extends well above the surface of the water to permit intake of air. We do not encourage patients to experiment! One of our patients became a salesman for outboard motorboats. While demonstrating a boat, he made too sharp a turn and fell out. Although he was removed quickly from the water, enough had entered his trachea to suffocate him. His friends knew nothing about first aid for laryngectomees.

say these things. Yet, for some patients this might be just the right approach. Hence, we insist that the surgeon prepare the patient for startling reactions (Howie; Pitkin). At the same time, he should give the patient assurance that his family will accept him, because he will be the same father and husband as he was before the operation. He need not fear that he will be unable to work; most laryngectomees of working age continue to work (Brodnitz; Gardner 1961, 1964; Horn). He will not lose his friends, his true friends; rather, they will praise his successes in learning to talk and in coming back to work (Gardner 1966). The surgeon should also caution the patient that much of his recovery of early capabilities will depend on his optimism, his determination and his desire to resume his normal living as soon as he leaves the hospital (Darley; McCall; McClear 1959; Schall 1954; Pitkin; Svane-Knudson).

The Family's Worries

Finally, we must not forget the patient's family. It is the surgeon's responsibility to orient them as well as the patient (Wintersteen). Gardner (1966) found that one-third of the husbands of prospective laryngectomized women were so upset that they were speechless. One husband remarked, "I can't take it. The strain is too great." Out of 235 couples where the wives were laryngectomized, two husbands divorced their wives; likewise 85 per cent of single women and 50 per cent of wives had no encouragement or advice from relatives while they were making up their minds to have surgery. One final point: The surgeon will be of great help to all concerned if he discusses how the patient can make it easier for his family. Andrews did this with a 12-year-old girl who was to be laryngectomized. She made it much easier for her mother, who was the one who had to be comforted.

ORIENTATION BY OTHERS

All of this information need not be thrown at the patient in one session. As stated above, the patient usually cannot take it all in at once. He must have time to meditate and to recover his equilibrium in order to ask questions sensibly and to make practical business and financial arrangements. The surgeon may be aided greatly if he calls upon allied professional persons to assist him in the orientation process (Brodnitz; Damsté; DiCarlo *et al.*; Ferguson; Gardner 1954; M.C.L. Greene; Hodson and Oswald; Jimison; Johannessen and Foy; Kusske; Lauder; Levin, Luchsinger and Arnold; McCall; McClear; Pitkin; Ranney; Wintersteen). He may call upon the psychologist to detect emotional difficulties and determine how they may be resolved. He may call upon local speech clinicians or former laryngectomized patients to make visits to prospective and postoperative patients. M.C.L. Greene advises:

> The patient will be greatly comforted if he can meet and speak with a proficient esophageal speaker. The laryngectomized, "cured" and successfully rehabilitated individual is able to demonstrate more convincingly than any other that life may go on with enjoyment and without too great inconvenience. He is able to describe from actual experience what laryngectomy means in terms of physical discomfort and personal, social and economic difficulties.

Wintersteen urges, "The presence of an intelligent, psychologically astute person can be a good support to the patient at this time."

Four different persons are available for the use of the surgeon in the preoperative or postoperative orientation of his patients. These are male and female laryngectomees, the wife of a male laryngectomee and the speech clinician. The laryngectomized visitants are selected from the membership of the Lost Chord Club because of their neat appearance, good speech and successful adjustments. The wife of a laryngectomee is a member of the Auxiliary of the club. She and her laryngectomized husband are known to have made satisfactory adjustments since his laryngectomy.* A call by the surgeon will receive a quick response from these people.

Visits by Male Laryngectomees

The male laryngectomee can demonstrate by his sheer presence that he has survived cancer, has learned to talk, has returned to work and is now present to help the patient to understand that he, too will succeed.†

Visits by Female Laryngectomees

The male laryngectomee commonly visits laryngectomized women because a female laryngectomee may not be available. However, the female laryngectomee is the preferred visitant to a female patient before or after laryngectomy. She will be neatly dressed with special care taken to cover her stoma and surgical scars with a clever scarf, thus appearing to dress like a person who has a larynx. She will have fluent esophageal speech and thus will show that she can communicate. She is proof that a woman who has cancer of the throat can survive and rise above her fears and no longer feel handicapped. She tells the patient to have confidence in her surgeon, to be cheerful to her husband and children and to look forward

---

* See the rules of conduct for visitants and how they are selected in Chapter 8.
† The actual conversation of the visiting laryngectomee will be found in Chapter 2.

to better health than she has at present. She replies to any questions about surgery by saying that the surgeon will answer them.

Wife-to-Wife Visits

With the consent of the surgeon, the wife of a laryngectomee endeavors to call on the wife of a man who is about to be laryngectomized. The patient's wife naturally may be greatly disturbed and confused over the news that her husband has cancer of the throat and must be operated on at once. Some wives appear outwardly calm but are inwardly shocked. Others weep copiously and cling to their husbands as if not to let them go. Their fears of cancer start a rush of anxious thoughts which deafen their ears to any assurances and explanations of the surgeon. It is this great need that impels the wives of laryngectomized husbands to help the anxious wife of a victim of cancer of the throat.

The visiting wife may meet the patient's wife at the surgeon's office, at the hospital bedside or in her home. In some instances it is only possible for her to call the patient's wife over the telephone. Martin (1963) has his secretary arrange for an older laryngectomee to telephone the office so that both the husband and wife can hear his esophageal voice and his words of assurance that the husband will be able to talk in the same way. Couples have been greatly comforted by this conversation.

If the visiting wife succeeds in having a person-to-person visit with the wife of a prospective laryngectomee, the following conversation has been found to be helpful in preparing the patient's wife for the unusual and unknown experiences that lie ahead: *

> "I am so glad that I can talk to you. My husband had the same operation, but I want to assure you that he is now talking, is back at work. I want very much to help you understand some of the things that all wives of laryngectomees go through. You know, it is not too bad for your husband to lose his larynx. He can't talk with it anymore because it is diseased and has to come out to save his life. He has the rest of his speech mechanism so that it should be only a short time until he will talk again.† Some husbands go to work shortly after they leave the hospital because the doctor says they are in good health. Others have problems that take longer; you understand that.
>
> I don't know how much the doctor told you, but I want to help you understand some things that might disturb you when you first see your husband after surgery. He will be bandaged around the head and neck. You will see a silver

---

* The conversation offered here is appropriate for the task of helping the patient's wife before surgery. An additional conversation will be offered later for the visit to the patient's wife after surgery. See Chapter 8 for more information on material to be given to the wife of a patient.

† This remark implies the possible use of the artificial larynx as an optional manner of recovering speech promptly. See Chapter 4 for information on the artificial larynx.

tube placed in a hole in his neck. He will breathe through that opening the rest of his life. It will be easier to breathe that way than the old way.

"He will cough a lot at first but this will diminish as his body gets accustomed to the new way of breathing. We barely notice anyone coughing at our club meetings. The nurse will show him how to draw up the mucus with an aspirator, a pumping machine. It's very noisy and may frighten you when you first hear it, but don't worry; it gives him quick relief. You will also see a vaporizer sending up steam near his head to keep his nose and throat moist. You will see a plastic tube in his nose that is used to feed him. In four or five days he can take food in his mouth and swallow it. The nurse will feed him at first, but he will soon be holding the bottle above his head to feed himself. It is wise to let him care for himself from the beginning so that he will not feel helpless or become dependent on you.

"While you are visiting him, you can help your husband feel more at ease by talking about what is going on at home, what mail came (let him read it if he wishes), what the children or relatives are doing and who called up to ask about him. Busy talk helps him to get reoriented to the homey things, and to forget the shock he went through and his present discomfort.

"Urge him to use a magic slate or scratch pad to communicate with you. If an artificial larynx has been lent to him, he should talk with it.* Both of you will know that the silent moments are over sooner than you expected.

"When the bandages are removed, don't show distress at the discoloration and the hole in the neck. He should begin to keep the opening covered by wearing a bib, especially when he expects visitors. Here's one that I made. The wives crochet their own for their husbands. The visitants will bring a package of some simple ones to wear right after surgery.

"Here is my card and telephone number. If you are worried about anything, call me at once. I will try to help you. If it's a medical question, call the doctor. He will be glad to help you if you are worried about something rather than let you stay anxious. I will talk to you again after your husband goes home."†

Visits by the Speech Clinician

The preoperative orientation is made more effective if a speech clinician is working in the hospital-clinic situation, where the surgeon may call upon him to help with the explanations that the patient needs (Heaver *et al.*; McClear 1959). He may cover some of the material the surgeon usually gives but with greater detail and with illustrative material about how a laryngectomized person will talk. He may show pictures of laryngectomees who are happily working on their jobs or are out golfing. M.C.L. Greene emphasizes the strong support given by the speech clinician:

* See Chapter 4.

† The question is often asked: "What about the husband of a laryngectomized wife?" This aspect has been neglected; hence, we are preparing a pamphlet that will include visitations not only by the wife of a laryngectomee but also by the husband of a laryngectomee, as well as by the laryngectomized male.

The speech pathologist by keeping in touch with the patient before and after operation pays out a life-line on which he can hold and the strength of which even the therapist may not fully realize.

Likewise, the speech pathologist can improve the relationship greatly by visiting the patient daily before and after surgery. He, as well as the surgeon, can thus spread out the information in smaller bits so that the patient can more easily absorb them and ask pointed questions.

Auditory and Visual Aids

The speech clinician may have at hand a motion picture that portrays the story of a man who had cancer of the larynx, had surgery and was completely rehabilitated. The surgeon or speech clinician may send the patient to a speech and hearing center to see such a film.*

The film story is most helpful because it vividly answers many questions, some of which the patient may not yet have considered. His recollection of scenes in the story during his immediate postoperative days may serve to maintain a higher morale. It is wise for relatives to see the film at the same time or later. Our record is nine relatives who witnessed the film with a father and grandfather who was to be operated on. This was a display of extraordinary family loyalty and concern.

The motion picture film story is an answer to the surgeons who protest against preoperative orientation. The patient who sees the laryngectomized actor and hears his voice in an average living situation will face the future with confidence. Brodnitz suggests using the recordings that accompany training records. They are long enough for the patient to determine in his own mind whether the esophageal speech is acceptable to him. Our experience with recordings of voices was not a happy one. In the temporary absence of a film projector, we substituted some disc recordings of former patients who had learned to talk. After the patient listened to them he said, "If I have to use a voice like that I will jump in the lake." Fortunately, he accepted surgery and later learned to talk. In contrast, one of our patients remarked after seeing the film, "I see now that everything will be OK for me, but just the same, I would prefer to keep my larynx."

Printed Information

In order to enable the patient to study questions and answers at leisure, the clinician may give him pamphlets which amply demonstrate that many

---

* The local or state units of the American Cancer Society have a selection of films on cancer of the larynx and rehabilitation of laryngectomees. Some of these are listed in the Appendix. It is also possible to show one film in the patient's hospital room. The film, *To Speak Again*, produced by Washington Hospital Center, Washington, D.C., is produced on an 8-mm cartridge for use with the Fairchild Projector. It may be obtained through the American Cancer Society.

others who had the same problem are enjoying life and are back at work. Much useful material is available through the International Association of Laryngectomees (IAL),* the national headquarters of 145 clubs located in many nations of the world. Some clubs have written and printed their own pamphlets that are also distributed to patients.

Presurgery Speech Instruction

Assurance that the laryngectomee will be able to speak after surgery has been one of the most important features of preoperative and postoperative programs of orientation. Supplementing the surgeon's assurance, the sound of the visitants' voices gives the patients the impression that speech recovery will be a routine procedure. We have heard laryngectomees tell a new member, "If you want to, you will learn to talk." This statement has been repeatedly offered by visitants and by speakers at IAL conventions, as well as at local club meetings. Some speech clinicians consider this remark to be too abrupt and a challenge to the patient's intentions.

Some surgeons, visitants and speech pathologists have gone beyond mere demonstrations. They have drilled the patients in initiating the esophageal sound before surgery (Berry and Eisenson; Gardner 1954; M.C.L. Greene; Loebell and Brahm; McCall; McClear 1959; Pitkin; Rickenberg; Snidecor; Waldrop and Baker). Snidecor says that the patient should "learn to charge air and perhaps vibrate the top of the gullet." After McClear obtains an initial speech sound during preoperative orientation, he says, "You have already taken the first step toward acquiring a new voice!" Some therapists (Gardner 1954; McClear 1959) have had the wife practice in getting the sound in order to assist and encourage the patient to practice.

M.C.L. Greene's preoperative preparation for speech is more extensive in that she gives the patient instructions in relaxation and central breathing in order to develop coordination of the respiratory and articulatory muscles. She believes that preliminary training in these activities brings earlier success in gaining fluency and synchronization of injection and aspiration of the air into the esophagus. It would thus appear that the early act of doing something constructive and practical about his voice problem would give the patient some reassurance. McCall states that delaying surgery for three or four days to instruct the patient in esophageal voice "greatly facilitates speech development." He reported that only three of nineteen patients who had no preoperative training in belching learned to use esophageal voice, whereas all thirteen of his patients who had preoperative voice training regained speech. In 1952, McCall and Fisher reported that 84 per cent of the ninety-nine patients who had preoperative training

---

* Founded by the author in 1952.

developed good or poor voices compared to 52 per cent of twenty-seven patients who obtained good or poor voices without it.

Citing McCall, Gardner and others who have taught belching before surgery, Martin (1963) stated:

> To me the proposition has always seemed of doubtful benefit and psychologi-cally unsound. I have never used it. . . . To the surgeon with insight and understanding of the psychological reaction of patients facing surgery for cancer of the larynx, it would seem unnecessarily crude and therapeutically harmful to direct a patient to go about belching while awaiting admission to the hospital and the journey to the operating room.

Shames *et al.* and Klieger found that presurgery instruction in speech did not always lead to proficiency in speech. Shames believes that the clinician's time and effort could be better directed toward counseling with the patient and his family on critical problems that occur prior to or following surgery. The patient's anxiety over coming surgery may have little value for post-operative speech success.

Levin (1955) has had his prospective and convalescent patients "sit in" on speech classes in order to get a psychological boost. We have very little information on the extent to which prospective laryngectomees are affected by seeing surgical scars and hearing the wheezing and coughing of laryngectomized patients who are learning to talk. Darley suggests that some fears of patients may be alleviated by practicing air intake preopera-tively. He thought that this may also give the patients an earlier start toward freeing themselves of pad and pencil. In our early clinical practice (Gardner 1961) we consistently urged the patient to practice swallowing with and without the use of carbonated water. Unfortunately the patients tried to do the swallow-belch while they were in the hospital and before they were released by the surgeon for speech therapy. This unforseen enthusiasm resulted in unexpected gastric disturbances. When the surgeons solved the mystery of several fistulas, they ordered cessation of preopera-tive training.

OVEROPTIMISM FOR SPEECH RECOVERY

Promising a preoperative or postoperative laryngectomized patient that he will talk again has been questioned (Diedrich and Youngstrom; Martin 1955, 1963), because it may raise false hopes if the patient eventually fails to acquire speech, if its acquisition is delayed for many months or if speech never becomes a suitable means of communication. Diedrich and Youngstrom assert that a visit to the patient by a laryngectomee who speaks well is no assurance that the patient will talk. Ample proof that promises of speech success are not justified for all patients is given by figures of successful acquisition of speech that range from 57 per cent to

75 per cent with an average of between 60 and 65 per cent (Gardner 1961; Heaver *et al.;* Horn; Johnson; Kindler; McCall and Fisher). Since as many as 40 per cent of the patients do not acquire esophageal speech, it would appear that a certain amount of deception is practiced on those patients who do not learn it. Heaver *et al.* stated that before surgery many of their patients thought they would speak again but that after surgery many of these same people lost their optimism about regaining their speech. In a panel discussion on the selection of a preoperative visitant, Andrews said:

> The selection of the proper laryngectomized person is, I think, a very important one. I think the patient should know how good speech can be, but we must realize that not every patient will learn to talk afterwards, and we should not misrepresent it by giving him the idea that everyone learns to speak and everyone learns to speak well, because I know that is not the case. There are all degrees of ability the same way as there are all degrees of ability in non-talking laryngectomized persons. . . . I happen to have some patients who use the mechanical larynx as well as esophageal speech, and I find it helpful with them because they demonstrate both methods of speaking.

Finally, Montreuil believes that failure to prepare a patient for the possibility that he will not acquire speech can result in a psychological setback.

Another interesting aspect of the promise of successful speech is the doubt among contemporary speech pathologists that they can obtain speech from all of their patients. They consider that preoperative training of a patient is truly idealistic. As college teachers, they regret that they themselves are unable to teach all of their speech pathology students to compress air for an esophageal speech sound; nor are they themselves all able to do what they require of a preoperative patient. The prospective laryngectomee may have doubts about eventually regaining his voice if his own speech clinician first explains the need for preoperative voice training and then fails to demonstrate his own esophageal voice. (Later we will discuss the role of the laryngectomee in this situation.)

Martin (1963) avoids misrepresentation by telling the patient that he will regain *adequate postlaryngectomy speech* by "one method or another." He makes sure that the patient fully understands that he will have some means of communication other than writing or whispering, that is, newly learned esophageal speech or communication by an artificial larynx, or both. (On this point, see also Luchsinger and Arnold, and Diedrich and Young-strom.) Some voice clinicians use part of the preoperative period to train the patient to speak with an artificial larynx. We believe it is wise even to show the spouse how easy it is to use an artificial larynx. After one of our patients had learned to speak with an instrument within a few minutes of practice, his mood changed from anxiety to great relief. He remarked, "I know I will be able to talk, but I still would like to keep my own voice."

Chapter Two

POSTLARYNGECTOMY ORIENTATION
OF THE PATIENT

THE PATIENT IN THE CONSTANT CARE ROOM

The period immediately following surgery is a very busy one for the patient. He lies in the constant care room where he receives the close attention of the staff. Attendants hover over him to take his temperature and blood pressure. A machine hums noisily as the nurse inserts an aspirator tube into his stoma to remove rapidly accumulating mucus. She feeds liquids through a plastic tube that enters his nose. Moist air is rising from a vaporizer beside his pillow. He is given medication to prevent infection. The patient soon realizes that he has gone through the surgery safely. He becomes aware of discomfort. His neck is terribly sore and he cannot swallow. He feels no air passing through his nose; he feels that he is breathing air through a hole somewhere in the bandages that bind his throat. When the nurses speak to him, all he can do is roll his eyes.

THE PATIENT IN THE HOSPITAL ROOM

After he returns from the constant care room to his nursing room, the patient is given a scratch pad and pencil so that he can tell the nurses how he feels and what he wishes. He may complain that he is hungry, which is a good sign. The patient shortly is able to leave his bed and walk. He looks at himself in the mirror. He sees the bandages around his head and neck and a silver tube protruding from his neck, through which he is breathing. He begins to think, and wonder and worry.

The Patient's Reaction to Surgery

A search of the literature reveals the many reactions that laryngectomees experience after they have survived surgery. Following is a condensation of the most commonly mentioned items:

1. Fears: death; recurrence of cancer; breathing problems; loss of smell, taste, voice, laughing, singing, whistling, sneezing.
2. Worries: inadequacy as a person because of mutilation and loss of body parts; cosmetic changes: scars, stoma or hole in the neck,

15

discoloration; loss of social acceptance; uselessness because of advancing age; lessening of earning power; loss of communication; loss of economic security; inability to care for family.

3. Emotional reactions: self-pity, guilt, resentment, disgust, depression, loneliness, thoughts of withdrawal from others.

Heaver *et al.* found that 32 of 274 patients displayed euphoric feelings prior to surgery in contrast to the others, who were depressed. After surgery, the number of patients with euphoria doubled. The euphoric reaction was explained as relief at the removal of the cancer.

A special study of the reactions of female laryngectomees finds agreement with the above summary (Gardner 1966). When they see their stomas for the first time, 48 per cent react unfavorably. They are horrified, shocked and disgusted. Some patients regard themselves as repulsive. Some say, "I'm a scarecrow. It's a blow to my vanity." Others react favorably by thinking, "Thank God I can breathe again" or "What a wonderful job of sewing me up!" Less than 35 per cent think that the scars and stomas make them less attractive to others, and about 23 per cent believe that surgery has made them less feminine. For these reasons, these women fear that their husbands will look to other women.

If the patient has had preoperative orientation, he may meet these thoughts with the reminder he was given: "Yes, they told me I would look like this, but I never dreamed it would be this bad. But I'm breathing and feeling better already. That's enough for me." Since investigators report that many patients become seriously depressed at this time, it is the appropriate time to have a visit from a laryngectomee, either for the first time or for the second time if the patient was visited prior to surgery (Gardner 1954, 1961; McCall; McCall and Stover; Pitkin; Schall). In 1941, Morrison quoted Stern as saying that a visit by a laryngectomee was a great help to the newly laryngectomized person. Damsté expressed the need for a visitor: "There is no one who is better able to encourage a patient than a man who has gone through the same predicament." Pitkin uses the visitant to build up the patient's morale and confidence by having him see someone who has survived surgery, has a good voice and bears testimony that complete rehabilitation is possible. He reported in 1953 that only one-third of the patients were visited by laryngectomees. From Horn's survey in 1960–61, we learned that 63 per cent of the patients had visitors, but only 3 per cent of those who were not visited would have preferred visits from laryngectomees.*

---

* It is rare in the Cleveland area for a patient not to be visited. The cooperation of the Lost Chord Club members and the surgeons is excellent. Some surgeons request visitations prior to surgery, but practically all of them request that laryngectomees visit the patients after surgery.

Postlaryngectomy Visits

Visits by the Patient's Wife

Sitting alone in his room, the patient contemplates the future. Did they get all of the cancer? Will it come back? How will he know? How soon can he go home? How soon can he return to work? Will they want him back at the shop? When the bandage is removed, he sees the hole in his neck, and the reddishblue scars. Perhaps he sees a sunken area where they resected muscle tissue from one side of the neck or he may notice that his shoulder is lower on that side.* He thinks, "I'm mutilated. I'll be deformed the rest of my life. What will Mary say when she sees me? What will the men say to me? I can't play golf any more. Maybe I can't even work."

When the patient sees his wife enter the room, his mind wants to say "Hello," but nothing happens. He thinks, "I can't say a word. I can't even speak to my wife. I can't smile." Belatedly, he greets her with a raised hand. He writes on the scratch pad that he is glad to see her, and asks how the children are; or he might write: "It's pretty rough!" Seeking sympathy, some patients write that they feel terrible (Gardner 1966). Others write that they are glad the "damned thing is out."

Visits by Male Laryngectomees

The surgeon calls the Lost Chord Club or the local speech and hearing center when he decides that the patient is ready for visitors. Upon his arrival, the visitant identifies himself and delivers a typical talk:

> "I am from the Lost Chord Club. Doc asked me to come to see you. I know just how you feel. I went through the same thing, but here I am telling you that you are going to come back just like the rest of us. I've brought a magic slate for you to write on. Just write with the wooden pencil and I can read it."

The patient may write: "I'm a dummy. I can't make a sound. I can't spit; I can't even sneeze." The visitor reads the writing and smiles as he says:

> "I understand all about that. You will be able to spit again. You will be able to talk again one way or another. Some fellows can sing, play a harmonica or a trumpet. Stop worrying right now. You'll soon be out of here and raring to start speech lessons, when the good doctor approves it. Here is an envelope of

---

* The castration complex is frequently mentioned in the literature (Diedrich and Young-strom; Moses; Pond). Pond, a laryngectomee, states that many of the patients he has visited or met at IAL meetings have told him that they have a feeling of amputation or "something cut out." He insists that they also have a "psychological amputation." He describes this as a momentary loss of both the mental and physical image of a word; in the middle of a sentence "it just drops out." For example, in the sentence, "I am going downtown," "down" may be blacked out completely. For a detailed description of deformities resulting from radical laryngectomies, read Norris.

bibs for you to use here in the hospital to cover your stoma when visitors come. The women at the American Cancer Society make them. Just tie the tapes back of your neck. You can get all kinds of bibs later on, fancy ones and plain ones that our wives make. Here is a book, *Helping Words*, that answers a lot of questions you have been worrying over. Here is another one, *Laryngectomees at Work*. It shows the many jobs that our members handle. These came from our national association, the IAL, which has 140 clubs throughout the world.

"Read these from cover to cover; have your wife and family read them, even your friends when they call on you. Here is our own pamphlet which greets you and tells how our club is ready to receive you and your wife to meet our members who meet once a month. After you go home, be sure to come and bring your wife with you. Here's my card. If you or your wife want to ask any questions, don't hesitate to call me. I'll be glad to come over as soon as you call."

The visitor must be brief and limit the visit to fifteen or twenty minutes (Kusske). He should show sympathy and understanding but must not tire the patient. An important rule is that he should not answer any questions of a medical or financial nature. It must be emphasized that he works according to rules agreed upon by the surgeons and the members of the local Lost Chord Club. (See the rules in Chapter 8.)

Wife-to-Wife Visits

About the time that the patient is ready to go home, the visiting wife makes a call in order to prepare the wife for problems that may arise at home. The following material may serve as a model of the type of information that wives have found to be important enough to give to the new wife.*

"When you have your husband back home, you will find that some readjustments are going to be necessary. The first thing to remember is that your husband must always be dressed neatly around the neck when friends come in. If any children are around, they should never see the bare neck. Be frank and tell them, if they ask, that your husband lost his voice box because it was diseased but that he will soon be able to talk in a different way. If he uses an artificial larynx, he can amuse the children by letting them talk with it. Everyone thus becomes relaxed and no one worries about his voice problem.

"I would like to suggest that pampering him is not good. Let him take care of his own stoma hygiene. Always have a supply of hankies or paper wipes handy so he can remove the mucus easily. Don't do it for him. If he wears a bib, he slips his hand under it to clear the mucus. If he wears a shirt, arrange to leave the button that is second from the top off the shirt or sew it on the

---

*The Auxiliary of the IAL has discussed these points at our national conventions, led originally by Mrs. Max Fried of the Detroit Anamilo Club. Some of the points that were discussed by Mrs. Fried are included in the presentation given here. Although it is written as a monologue, the visit may consist of questions and answers.

outside of the buttonhole. He then can reach through and wipe the mucus from beneath the bib and shirt. You can get crocheted bibs from the women in the club or make some yourself. We'll show you how. You even can match the bibs with the color of the shirt. You may look through this book of patterns of scarves and covers that both men and women use to dress attractively.†

"Be sure to have him attend the first meeting of our Lost Chord Club. Give him the impression that you take it for granted he will go, and stick with it. He will see many others who had the same operation and are now happily back with their friends and families. And be sure to keep him going to speech class both with his teacher and at the club. The members will encourage him and be glad to help him.

"If you and your husband are in a group, don't hesitate to tell strangers that he had his voice box removed, but that he can hear well, so talk naturally to him. An early explanation to a hostess will prevent all kinds of embarrassments.

"Urge him to go out by himself. Send him on errands so he can meet people. These activities will make him happy and keep him busy. Be sure to urge him to use the words he has learned. Sooner or later you will want to urge him to talk to you with words, then phrases and finally sentences.* Here is my card. Be sure to call me if anything goes wrong. I will be glad to talk to you or to come over and bring my husband."

Visits by Female Laryngectomees

It is extremely desirable that a female laryngectomee visit the newly laryngectomized female. She should be neatly dressed, and her stoma should be covered by an attractive scarf or jeweled piece, or a high-necked dress (Fig. 1). She explains the purpose of her visit as already presented above. In addition, she tells the patient:

"Don't worry about loss of attractiveness; we laryngectomized women have learned to maintain our charm and femininity. Don't fear that you have lost the love and attention of your husband. If he was devoted to you before surgery, he will be the same to you now, and the children will love you just the same. But be sure always to dress neatly so that no one ever sees the scars or the opening in your neck. You must not permit feelings of bitterness or loneliness to disturb you. I was worried about gaining weight more than anything else! If you worked before, you will work again. If you had a lot of friends, they will be anxious to have you back with them. It takes courage and patience and determination to regain the things that you think you have lost. Here are pictures of some of our women laryngectomees. See how beautifully they are dressed? We have worked out all kinds of patterns for bibs, scarves and special dress arrangements and now have them in this pamphlet. We also have workshops to design our own patterns of jewelry. I'll be seeing you at the next club meeting. Here's my card. Call me if you have any questions or problems."

† Available through the IAL.

* Of course, if he uses the artificial larynx, he will be talking much sooner. However, he still should be encouraged to continue with speech lessons, and he should have training on the proper use of the instrument.

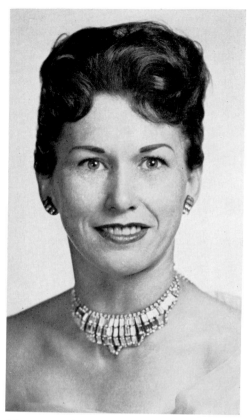

Figure 1. Jeweled necklace worn by a laryngectomee. (*Courtesy of American Medical Association*)

COMMUNICATION PROBLEMS OF THE LARYNGECTOMEE

In the first postoperative days, the nurses and surgeons have difficulty obtaining information about how the patient feels and what he wants. He may use a magic slate or a scratch pad but this is slow and frustrating to both parties. The patient lies helplessly while his family talks about what is going on at home or at the office. If his business associates come to see him, he is fearful that they will think something besides his speech is wrong with him. Likewise, the illiterate person who can neither read nor write cannot communicate except by signs. These problems can be quickly solved by lending every laryngectomized patient an artificial larynx (Diedrich and Youngstrom). The foreign language problem may be solved by having a hospital employee or some friend with the same language background interpret the patient's message, or the spouse might know English well enough to be of help. In addition, speech clinicians are accustomed to preparing cards for various types of patients, such as aphasic persons, which may be pointed to by the patient to indicate what he wants.

The Patient's Need for an Artificial Larynx

Martin (1963) explains the need for giving laryngectomees a speaking appliance as soon as it is medically safe:

> In most discussions on speech rehabilitation, one may search in vain for any consideration or even mention of one obviously simple fact, to wit: that to one suddenly deprived of the capacity for a means of audible communication, . . . that specific method of artificial speech should be used immediately which will most quickly enable the patient to communicate audibly again with medical attendants, family, employers, and business associates. At this point, it may be stated unequivocally that the use of a mechanical sound-producing device is the only means by which artificial speech can be restored within a few days after operation in all cases.

Because of the massive bandages wrapped around the neck and head of the patient, the only usuable styles of artificial larynx for this purpose are those with which vibrations are introduced to the mouth. One of these types is an electronic larynx which transmits vibrations through a plastic tube to the mouth, where they are modified for speech sounds. Another is a pneumatic type which receives stoma air at one end and transmits the vibrated air at the other end, which is inserted into the mouth. According to Irwin, the Lost Chord Club of Memphis lends a Cooper-Rand Electronic Larynx to each patient while he is in the hospital at the University of Memphis Medical Center. The laryngologists not only approve of this procedure, but one of them donated six aids for use by the club. Other suitable models will be also presented and discussed in Chapter 4.

Putting an artificial speech aid in the hands of a laryngectomee so early in the postoperative period (or at any later time) may not be acceptable to some surgeons who firmly oppose the use of any mechanical instrument. Hence, this helpful procedure may only be practiced when the local Lost Chord Club members, the speech clinicians and the surgeons agree with this policy.

Our first experience with a homemade instrument that transmitted vibrations into the mouth gave fascinating proof of its value in the postoperative period:

> A male patient was lying in his bed on the sixth postoperative day. After receiving the surgeon's permission, we introduced ourselves to the patient and explained that we wished to demonstrate to him that he would always be able to communicate by some kind of speech. After showing him how to hold the end of the flexible cup tightly over his stoma and to insert the other end of the

tube into his mouth, we asked him to whisper *one-two-three*. A very audible speech came forth, much to the patient's surprise. Shortly after we had been practicing talking, the patient's brother entered the room. We told the patient to say, "Hi, Ed" with the tube. The sober countenance of the brother changed to a grin of surprise and delight. The patient's wife entered. He greeted her with "Hi, Mary." She stood motionless, opened her mouth, put her handkerchief to her eye, then quickly recovering, smiled and exclaimed, "Why Fred, you can talk!" He replied, "You bet I can."*

We had more difficulty with a second patient who was unable to read or write. The surgeon wanted to ask him some questions. We had him use the Cooper-Rand Electronic Larynx, but we could not understand him. We discovered why: he did not have any teeth! It is sufficient to say here that any patient's frustrating, depressing moment may be quickly replaced with understanding and hope for adequate communication with all of its rewards.

* The homemade instrument used during this experiment is shown in Figure 6 (page 56).

Chapter Three

PLANNING THE LARYNGECTOMEE'S
REHABILITATION

RESPONSIBILITY OF THE SURGEON

By the time the laryngectomee is ready to leave the hospital, the surgeon either will have begun to prepare for the patient's future or will at this time take definite steps in this direction. Writers (Holinger *et al.;* Loebell and Brahm; Martin 1963) have repeatedly asserted that the surgeon who takes away the patient's ability to talk, which in turn deprives him of the ability to make a living, has the responsibility of restoring the patient to his original status. Fulfillment of this responsibility involves the following measures: (a) planning for continued improvement of the patient's physical condition and comfort; (b) planning for faithful follow-up visits by the patient; (c) counseling or recommending counseling on reemployment and on the psychological, economic and social aspects of the patient's rehabilitation; (d) advising the patient to join the local or nearest Lost Chord Club; and (e) initiating speech therapy through referral.

Physical Conditions and Comfort

Discharge from the hospital and the return home can be a critical event for the laryngectomized patient. This is especially true when no attempt is made to train the patient in proper self-care. Most surgeons delegate to the nursing staff the demonstration of aspiration, removal and cleansing of the tracheal tube cannula (inner tube), sterilization and reinsertion. Everything is explained, including proper washing of the hands, and careful handling of the tube, aspiration catheter and nasal suction. As soon as he is physically capable, the patient (under nursing supervision) begins to perform these necessary chores by himself. When the tracheal tube itself is to be replaced, the surgeon or a member of the hospital staff demonstrates its removal and reinsertion, and explains the reasons why it is important for the patient to learn the correct procedure. This participation by the patient in his own postoperative care not only prepares him for home self-care but stabilizes him psychologically by keeping him busy during his trying postoperative period, thus leading him gradually to a feeling of self-confidence in dealing with the problems of his newly altered anatomy. During this time, the spouse visiting at the bedside participates in these instructions and demonstrations and is particularly instructed to encourage and assist the patient.

Mucus

One of the most important (and potentially most serious) problems is that of excessive mucus production in the trachea. This is greatest in the immediate postoperative period when the patient has not regained full consciousness and constant suction-aspiration is necessary to keep a clean tracheal airway. The sudden change from nasal to "neck" breathing leads to excessive mucus production in the trachea. The added effects of surgery on the delicate sensitive lining of the trachea, plus the presence of the tracheal tube itself, stimulate excessive mucus production.* At this time, the presence of an active cough reflex (although aggravating to the patient and his family) protects the patient from serious lung complications. Pekarek cautions that *no cough-suppressing drugs* should be administered during this period for that very reason.†

The family is encouraged by being told that this excessive mucus production will gradually abate as the trachea becomes accustomed to the "raw" atmosphere.‡ However, it must be understood that a certain amount of mucus secretion must always be present in the tracheobronchial tree, just as the nose and mouth, bladder and intestinal tracts must be kept moist constantly, if they are to function properly. Hence, the problem is not one of elimination but of control.

Humidity

It is considered ideal for a laryngectomee to live in an atmosphere with a relative humidity between 35 and 50 per cent, and with an air temperature of 50 F to 75 F. Individual variations and preferences vary so greatly that it is impossible to make any hard and fast rules. Dr. Pekarek describes his personal experience with a mucus problem:

> Let us clarify the situation by a true example. While travelling to the west coast for an I.A.L. convention, a driver was accompanied by a fellow laryngectomee, who at all times complained of excessive mucus production. When they drove through Nevada and Arizona, the companion confided that for the first time, he experienced complete relief from tracheal mucus. He felt

---

* Some surgeons recommend that the patient rent a suction device from a local medical supply house when he goes home. Some clubs lend them to their members.

† V. F. Pekarek, MD, a laryngectomized surgeon, is Medical Adviser to the Cleveland Lost Chord Club and Co-Chairman of the Committee on First Aid and Safety of the IAL.

‡ Reed states that the mucosa undergoes metaplasia to a squamous type of epithelium. It then will be compatible with the dry air that is no longer being moistened by the nose.

"just fine." On the other hand, the driver could hardly wait for privacy to manually remove hard, tracheal mucus crusts. He was miserable in spite of moistening his bibs with water. In retrospect, he believes that an air-conditioner in his car would have helped him.

Proper humidification, especially during the cold winter weather, is helpful. Dr. Pekarek uses two humidifiers. In nonwinter months, ordinarily he uses an Emerson humidifier. He runs it from 6:00 or 7:00 in the evening until bedtime, then shuts it off (with closed doors, of course). If the air is particularly dry, he runs it all night. In zero weather, he uses a Walton humidifier. It is a cold steam type which will peel off the wallpaper in the room if it is left on too long.

Incrustation

Incrustation around and within the trachea near the opening is somewhat similar to mucus that becomes dried within the nostril. As it is a product of dryness, control of the moisture content of the environment is of first importance in preventing its occurrence. However, many laryngectomees (89 per cent according to Diedrich and Youngstrom) admitted that they had the problem. In our experience, the problem has become so serious with some patients that they have had to be rushed to the laryngologist for emergency removal of the crusts.

Laryngectomees report several methods for removing the crusts from the stoma. Saline solution is most commonly mentioned, but others are steam, atomizer spray, petroleum jelly and even peroxide (Diedrich and Youngstrom). The patients should be cautioned about the use of such materials, using only what the surgeon recommends. Another dangerous habit is the use of cotton tips or pieces of loose cotton. Only a slight inward movement of air may cause aspiration of foreign matter. Some patients report that they tie a fishline around the tweezers or applicators as a precaution (Diedrich and Youngstrom). Wives have become adept at removing the crusts.

Coughing

During the first year after laryngectomy, coughing is a problem and an embarrassment with all laryngectomees because of its inconvenience and frequency. Horn reported that 58 per cent were coughing at the time of his survey; Diedrich and Youngstrom stated that 99 per cent admitted coughing had been a problem, and 40 per cent continued to be bothered. With careful hygiene under the surgeon's supervision and through his instructions, the coughing should decrease rapidly in succeeding months. In a typical group of laryngectomees, coughing is not any more noticeable than it is in an audience of normal persons. One only hears an occasional cough.

Having associated with laryngectomees for thirty years, we have observed their habits of cleaning out the mucus before they leave their room, and repeating the operation as soon as they return. They manage to avoid coughing while they are associating with others. If it is necessary to cough, they usually do it quietly and merely cough against the stoma cover. This additional moisture helps maintain a moist, warm environment for the edges of the stoma. Mixed with air, the mucus dissolves quickly. If the cougher prefers to remove the mucus, he slips his handkerchief under the collar where the shirt is left open at the second button.

Stoma Guards and Covers

Stoma guards (Fig. 2) are used by laryngectomees because cloth bibs tend to be sucked against the stoma by inhalation. As a result, the patients

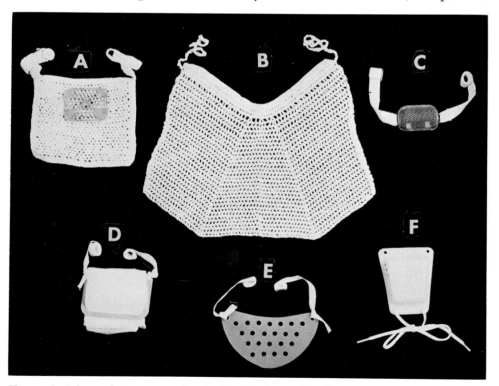

Figure 2. Bibs and stoma guards. *A*. McClear's crocheted stoma bib with detachable stoma guard. *B*. Oversized crocheted bib of nylon. *C*. Kenloc stoma guard. (Kenneth Lockwood). *D*. Stamped aluminum frame with gauze cover (United Surgical Company). *E*. Homemade punched plastic stoma guard. *F*. Molded plastic stoma guard (ABA Surgical Company). (*Courtesy of American Medical Association*)

feel that their air supply is reduced. Perforated stoma guards of different styles and makes may be worn between the stoma and the bib. When the patients become well adjusted to their new physical problems, they often discard the stoma guard.

Stoma covers, popularly called bibs (Fig. 2), are used to cover the stoma. Visitants give the hospital patients bibs made by the volunteers of the American Cancer Society.* Later, patients buy crocheted bibs from the Auxiliaries of the clubs or their wives make them. Various types of material are used for changes in weather and for protection from harmful substances in the many kinds of industries that employ laryngectomees. Women can take special advantage of their femininity to use many kinds of attractive materials.†

Discontinuing Use of the Tracheal Tube

If the patient is to continue to use a tracheotomy tube temporarily or permanently (many now leave the hospital without a tube), he must wear it according to the surgeon's directions. He must keep it in at all times or at prescribed periods during the day or night. Patients who have disregarded these instructions have been rushed to emergency wards when the tubes were left out too long and the stoma opening shrank. The surgeon decides when the patient stops using the tube. Johnson states that thirty-one of the patients operated on at a Veterans Administration hospital wear the tube permanently. The surgeon or staff member will explain to the patient how important it is for him to observe the surgeon's follow-up program.

Protecting the Stoma from Water During Showers

Several procedures are mentioned by the surgeon regarding taking care of the stoma during showers. A most simple method is to fold a washcloth into a square and hold it over the stoma while cleansing the body with the other hand. A shower shield (Fig. 3) is also available. One can breathe from the bottom of the shield without water entering the stoma. Another suggestion is to have the shower head placed lower so that the water strikes the lowest part of the body.

It is wiser still to take a tub bath so that less water is hurtling at the body. Under these conditions, it is advisable always to have a tub mat in order to insure good footing getting in and out, and to hold on to a

* The Cleveland unit of the American Cancer Society has three centers where patients may obtain bibs, as well as the usual supplies for cancer patients.

† For an extensive description of bib designs and materials for all kinds of wear, consult Diedrich and Youngstrom; and Gardner 1961, 1964, 1966. Also inspect the booklet of bib designs published by Sals (laryngectomized women) of the IAL, from which it may be purchased.

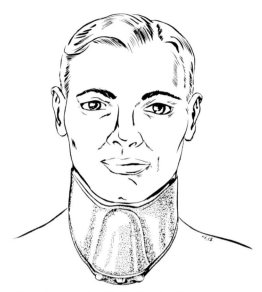

Figure 3. Rubber molded shower shield (C.L. Sheldon). (*Courtesy of American Medical Association*)

wall handle if there is one. McClear advises putting a face towel around the neck so that perspiration accumulating during the bath does not enter the stoma. He even advises avoiding strongly perfumed soaps which may irritate the stoma area. Many people are allergic to ingredients used in scented soaps (McClear 1969).

Frequent Follow-up Programs

The surgeon outlines a schedule of appointments for return visits. He warns the patient that promptness and faithfulness in observing the appointment dates are most important. The schedule must be followed over a period of five years, at which time it is considered that the cancer has been cured (McCall). The patient must be alert to any changes, such as lumps, irritations or bleeding around his stoma and in the area of the neck. It is important that he return to the surgeon at once when he notices any change. Otherwise, misfortune may come to him, as it did in the following tragedy of neglect.

A patient had been told that he had cancer of the larynx and surgery was planned, but he procrastinated for four months before returning for the laryngectomy. He later neglected the regular checkups. Five months later he returned because a lump had appeared on the same side of the neck on which he had been operated. Told that it must be removed at once, he went home and delayed returning for another four months. The ultimate result of this neglect was predictable.

Some patients may never return to the surgeon for checkups, if they were originally referred to him by a distant physician. In this situation, the surgeon sends the patient back to the local physician with instructions for care of the physical problems. The local doctor should assume the important task of counseling the patient on his economic and emotional problems and on communication aspects of his altered physical condition. It is his responsibility to call up proper professional persons or agencies to resolve any problems that may develop.

Since the patient usually returns for reexamination over a period of five years (McCall), the surgeon has frequent opportunities to ascertain any changes in his physical, emotional or communicative status (Martin 1963). Members of the family may report problems to the physician. If serious mood changes are evident, he should refer the patient to a social service center. If the patient is not using oral communication and has no artificial larynx as a substitute, the surgeon should first search for any physical reasons for the failure to communicate before discussing the problem with the speech clinician.

Counseling the Patient

The patient will be anxious to know when he can return to work. The surgeon may give an approximate date or may urge him to take it easy and not be in a hurry to go back; much depends on the patient's physical and emotional condition. If the patient is physically and emotionally sound, the surgeon can ask him whether his company has retained an opening for his return. If the answer is negative, the surgeon may inquire personally, or have a business friend inquire, about the reasons. He may consult with the company's personnel officer, the patient's immediate foreman or the supervising staff regarding the employee's status.*

If the surgeon is told that specific work conditions might create a health hazard, he should urge the company to employ the patient in another department where that hazard does not exist. The local Bureau of Vocational Rehabilitation may be asked to determine the feasibility of reemployment or of training in other specialties. The important point to emphasize is that although some patients may have a weakened arm from excessive loss of tissue, laryngectomees, as a whole, are generally sound in all respects except that they do not have a voice box.

* See Chapter 8 for further plans for assisting in reemployment. Additional employment problems are discussed in Gardner 1966.

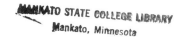

The Patient's Emotional Status

During the later days of the patient's stay in the hospital, the surgeon's daily visits will permit him to evaluate the patient's moods and morale. He may assume that the patient's own powers of recuperation, aided by visitants from the Lost Chord Club and from the family, should naturally restore his optimism and buoyancy. M. C. L. Greene believes that individual personal relationships with the nurses, surgeons, family and friends can impede or hasten rehabilitation. The surgeon should detect the absence of expected improvements in mood. In fact, he may be able to contrast the patient's attitudes as they were before surgery with the latest status. The surgeon may have already been forewarned of trouble, especially if the patient is an alcoholic, drug addict or diabetic or has a typical depressive type of personality. Gastric or duodenal ulcers may have been aggravated by the sudden physiological changes, which have exposed the patient's stomach to excessive quantities of air. These possibilities must be taken into consideration in regard to the ultimate discharge of the patient, which may be delayed for prescribed physical, psychiatric or social service studies and guidance. This service is conveniently obtained if the patient is in a hospital-clinic center. (Johannessen and Foy). Otherwise, the physician must refer the patient to services that are available nearby.

Joining the Lost Chord Club

The surgeon should emphasize the importance of the patient and spouse attending Lost Chord Club meetings. He may remark:

> "You will meet many people who have had a laryngectomy, both men and women. You will notice that they are having a good time, just like the person with a larynx. You will also notice that they are talking and smiling. They will be glad to welcome you, and their wives will offer to help your wife with the questions that always come up when a laryngectomee goes home from the hospital. Don't forget to go. Here's a card to remind you; it's on the last Friday of the month."

The surgeon or speech clinician may show pictures of a national meeting of IAL or of other persons who are having a good time at a social gathering. With the men neatly dressed with formal shirts and ties and the women with scarves around their necks, it is impossible to suspect that they have holes in their necks!

Referral for Speech Therapy

The surgeon's responsibility includes guidance of the patient concerning speech therapy (Brodnitz; Diedrich and Youngstrom; Gardner 1966; Gilmore; Loebell and Brahm; Martin 1963; Montreuil; Morrison 1941; Nahum and Golden; Norris). Some surgeons have assumed the task of instructing their patients in the production of esophageal speech (Levin 1965; McCall; Orton). Other surgeons do nothing about speech therapy referral. Forty-seven per cent of Diedrich and Youngstrom's patients were given no plans for speech therapy. We still find silent laryngectomees or poor speakers who apparently were not guided to a speech therapist, a procedure that should be routine. Since it is the duty of the surgeon to initiate the program for speech therapy, he may request his secretary to make the appointment for the patient.

Financial limitations should not cause a delay in obtaining speech therapy; many local units or state divisions of the American Cancer Society furnish funds for free instruction. The local office of the Bureau of Vocational Rehabilitation may arrange training for patients who are referred to them for reemployment. With all of these supporting services available, there need be no cause for anyone not receiving therapy. When this happens, however, we cannot always lay the blame on the surgeon. Unfortunately, some patients do not have the drive and determination to keep speech appointments or to persist in practicing. Still others avoid all contact with would-be benefactors and live on whatever funds they can obtain from relief agencies or from the Social Security Administration.

RESPONSIBILITY OF THE SPEECH CLINICIAN

While he is training the patient in esophageal speech, the speech clinician should assume the responsibility of urging the patient to attend the meetings of the local Lost Chord Club. This will serve as an inspiration for the laryngectomee to continue with speech therapy and to begin communicating with members of the club in his limited way. It is important to urge the spouse to go with the patient to the club, not only to insure that he will get there, but also to benefit from the interchange of ideas with other spouses.

From our personal experiences with programs of voice therapy for laryngectomees, and from conversations with other speech clinicians, we know that some of the latter participate heavily in counseling and rehabilitation of laryngectomees simply because no one else has assumed the task. It is fortunate for the patient if his speech clinician has a background in psychosocial aid to the handicapped. Regarding this point, Snidecor (1968) says:

> It is also to be noted that the speech pathologist will, in all probability, have psychological training so that he may counsel with both the laryngectomized individual and family members. He also may be in a very favorable posi-

tion of going "to bat" for the laryngectomee with his employer. The nature of the operation can be explained to the employer, and it can be noted that speech, if once established, will gradually become more fluent and intelligible. Emphasis can be given to the fact that the individual remains physically and intellectually capable, and that he may be even more motivated than he had been in the past.

If the speech clinician does not have the background just discussed, he should use the local welfare service, the speech and hearing center and other professional services whenever they are needed. Since he works frequently with the patient, he is in a good position to detect problems. Confidential talks with the spouse are helpful in uncovering difficult situations. It is not infrequent to find that alcohol is in the picture. The speech clinician should always report his suspicions or findings to the referring surgeon, if these problems appear to be delaying early re-adjustment.

We must give a word of caution here: No one who is not trained in clinical psychology or psychotherapy should attempt to advise a patient on emotional problems, let alone on more serious ones. However, our experience with voice patients of all kinds is that good, intense speech therapy, designed to give insight and understanding, and given in an enthusiastic, cheerful manner by a devoted teacher, has enabled many patients to make satisfactory adjustments to their emotional and social difficulties.

Chapter Four

BASES FOR POSTLARYNGECTOMY SPEECH

ANATOMICAL CHANGES AFFECTING THE SPEECH
OF LARYNGECTOMEES

The anatomical changes that are produced by a simple laryngectomy emanate from the removal of the larynx and/or surrounding tissues. The outstanding result of this surgery is the severance of the larynx from the trachea below and from the hypopharynx above. The latter now serves only as the pathway for food and liquids from the mouth into the esophagus. Pulmonary air can no longer enter the pharynx and mouth, nor can the patient breathe air through his mouth into his lungs. The open (cephalad) end of the trachea (severed from the larynx) is sewed to the outer skin at the front of the neck. This opening or tracheal stoma permanently serves for the ingress and egress of air from the lungs.*

Removal of the larynx makes necessary repair of the area around the junction of the esophagus with the hypopharynx. At this area, called by Decroix *et al.* the *pharyngo-esophageal* (PE) *junction or segment,* is the site of the pseudoglottis or, as Diedrich and Youngstrom call it, the *neoglottis,* the opening of the segment that leads into the hypopharynx. In the area of this segment may remain portions of the original fibers of the cricopharyngeal sphincter and/or the inferior fibers of the inferior pharyngeal constrictor muscles (hypopharynx). If some of the voluntary contractile fibers remain within the PE segment, the usual tonic sphincter-like closure may continue to function. The upper one-third of the esophagus is the site of the air chamber into which the oral-pharyngeal air is injected through the neoglottis and from which the air is ejected into the pharynx for voice production. It is interesting that the neoglottis, which survives as the vibratory or generating source of power for voice production, is located at about the same vertebral level as the original larynx and its glottis (Damsté; Moolenaar-Bijl 1953a).†

When the cancer has spread beyond the patient's larynx, the surgeon may excise adjoining parts that are involved. In addition to total laryn-

---

* For detailed information on the laryngectomy and its anatomical changes consult Diedrich and Youngstrom; Levin 1962; Norris; Snidecor 1968; and ear, nose and throat texts.

† See Diedrich and Youngstrom for a discussion of the various levels which may be the site of a neoglottis. See also Figure 12 of this book.

gectomy, a radical neck dissection may be performed, unilaterally or bilaterally, depending on how the cancer has spread (metastasis). This is done routinely by some surgeons because their pathologists so often find lymph nodes of the neck infiltrated with cancer cells.† The surgeons may remove a block of tissue that includes some of the accessory breathing muscles, nerve fibers, the external carotid artery and in some cases some shoulder muscles, hoping to take along with them all of the nodules which may have become involved. Metastasis may also involve the walls of the hypopharynx, the posterior and basal portions of the tongue, the entire tongue, the floor of the mouth and part of the jaw, as well as the upper third of the esophagus (Levin 1962; Snidecor 1968).

Radiation may be given as a curative therapy in lieu of surgery or it may be given postoperatively as supplementary insurance or as a palliative (Ogura). In either case, the flexibility of the irradiated tissues varies with the strength and duration of the treatment and may contribute to an unsatisfactory esophageal voice (Damsté; Diedrich and Youngstrom).

PHYSIOLOGICAL CHANGES AFFECTING THE SPEECH OF LARYNGECTOMEES

The outstanding changes in the laryngectomee's speech complex are the loss of the larynx as a vibrator and the disconnection of the pulmonary air column that supplied air for the articulatory function in the pharyngeal and oral cavities. Pulmonary air now passes outward through the new opening or stoma in the neck. Although the PE segment, the mouth of which is the new vibrator or neoglottis, is approximately at the same level as the excised larynx, that is, between the upper third of the esophagus and the inferior pharyngeal muscle,* it cannot be activated by pulmonary air. Nor can vibrating air, normally emanating from the larynx, be modified by the pharyngeal and oral structures. This means that the driving pressures for speech production that are developed primarily by the respiratory musculature and that normally pass through the trachea into the narrowed larynx, thence into the pharynx and mouth, are no longer available for an esophageal speaker.

UTILIZING THE RESIDUAL SPEECH MECHANISM

Loss of the tracheal air supply is a genuine and serious handicap to the laryngectomee's attempt to communicate. However, much of the speech mechanism remains to be utilized by the patient:

† Reports from Division of Pathology, Cleveland Clinic Foundation, to surgical staff.

* Descriptions of other possible locations for a pseudoglottis which might serve as an optional constriction area may be found in Damsté; and Diedrich and Youngstrom.

1. The laryngectomee must use a different source of air supply. This new supply is the air that is always present in the pharyngeal and oral cavities, as well as air that may necessarily be taken in through the mouth or possibly through the nasopharynx if the soft palate is relaxed.

2. The laryngectomee must utilize a different medium for receiving charged or injected air, that is, air that is compressed and moved into the esophageal air chamber. Since compression can best be made within a closed cavity (Diedrich and Youngstrom), the oral lips must be closed and the nasal pharynx must be sealed off from the oral pharynx by the soft palate (Damsté; Stetson). In this dynamic situation, the one flexible opening that is available for influence by compression or movement of air air within the oral and pharyngeal cavities is the space within the tonically contracted PE segment. Fortunately, the strength of the original crico- pharyngeal muscular contraction is usually somewhat reduced by surgery (Bateman and Negus; van den Berg *et al.;* Brighton and Boone; Damsté; Diedrich and Youngstrom; M.C.L. Greene). The neoglottis may be opened by the greater air pressure developed above it within the oral and pharyngeal cavities. Several media are available for trapping and moving air into the esophagus. These are the tongue, lips, cheeks, floor of the mouth and soft palate. The air also may be drawn (sucked) directly into the esophagus by inhalation (Damsté; Diedrich and Youngstrom; Snidecor 1968). More details on these movements will be found later in this chapter.

3. The laryngectomee must develop the ability to expel air back upward from the esophagus to generate air pressure waves that will be modified by the tongue, lips and teeth (Damsté 1957, 1958; Diedrich and Young- strom).* Since the respiratory mechanism is still intact, it is available for developing positive and negative pressures within the esophagus that will contribute to the new method of air intake and expulsion. Inherent char- acteristic tissue actions and reactions to stimuli and pressures will also serve the same purpose. The mechanism of expulsion will be discussed later in this chapter.†

4. The laryngectomee must learn to utilize the moving column of air that is expelled from the esophagus, as well as air in the oral and pharyn- geal cavities that may not have been injected during the air charge (Diedrich and Youngstrom). The patient first uses his lips, cheeks and tongue (with the soft palate closed) to compress the oral and pharyngeal

---

* For a vivid description of the expulsive action, see van den Berg *et al.;* Damsté 1958; and Snidecor 1968.

† There are other changes, such as changes in cavity size, temporal factors and pressure factors, but these need not be presented here for the purpose of training patients and students. Speech pathologists will wish to refer to van den Berg *et al.;* Damsté; Diedrich and Young- strom; and Snidecor 1968.

air and move it backward into the esophageal reservoir. He may merely inhale or may draw air into the esophagus as well. He next must eject or expel the air from the esophagus into the resonance areas, the pharyngeal and oral cavities. The air set into vibration within the neoglottis is the voiced sound that is modified into vowels and consonants by the same articulators that compressed the air. A certain amount of the air that is still within the oral-pharyngeal cavities may also be compressed for production of the voiceless consonants.

We must emphasize that the patient's tongue now performs a dual function, compression of air into the esophagus and, immediately after the air has been expelled, consonant-vowel production. The patient takes ½ second to inject air into the esophagus (Berlin 1965a; Damsté; Diedrich and Youngstrom; Snidecor and Curry). About ⅕ second later he ejects the air into the pharynx and oral cavities where he uses it for forming vowels and consonants. Of course, the tongue does not do double duty when the patient inhales air directly into the esophagus because it is first kept immobile to permit the free flow of air. Thus, the atmospheric air at the supraglottic level is ready to be moved in when the neoglottis relaxes. The fact is that the dual action of the tongue takes place so quickly and in such rapid sequence that it should be regarded as a single, whole action (Damsté; Diedrich and Youngstrom; Stetson 1937a). It is indeed remarkable how adaptable the human brain and its organs are; the laryngectomee is capable of developing one or more methods of taking air in differently from normal persons, and of quickly utilizing the same activators to produce esophageal speech.

HOW IS ARTICULATION ALTERED?

In the early days of therapy for esophageal speech, less attention was paid to the production of consonants than to the production of vowels (voice). We first believed that developing the esophageal sound was sufficient, and that the consonants would take care of themselves. Kallen stated that the patient "readily learns voiced and unvoiced consonants." Darley (1963) said that the vibrator produces sound which is "shaped in the conventional way by the articulators to form intelligible speech." M.C.L. Greene said, "Once voice is mastered, the patient can speak since there is no impairment of the organs of articulation." Wepman *et al.* stated: "Only the ability to produce sound is affected by the removal of the source of sound production, the larynx producing thereby a lack of communication between the body of air in the lungs and the articulators." Diedrich and Youngstrom stated that Stetson "did not view articulation in the laryngectomee as different from normal speech. . . ." Finally, Hodson and Oswald said that they "merely tell the patients to pronounce the various consonants in the way they have always done."

Our continued experience with patients has shown us that the above assumptions were not wholly true. We noticed that some patients did not pronounce the final consonants of a word or a phrase, and dropped or whispered the final word or syllable of a sentence. Some consonants were pronounced more easily than others. These deviations surely indicate that a patient has articulatory problems. Hence, we favored using the easy sounds and syllables in our therapy to help the patient learn the hard ones.

We also were puzzled when an occasional patient would be able to say a long phrase or sentence without pausing for frequent air intakes, but then would have great difficulty with the next phrase or sentence. So we rehearsed the patient with the easier sentences and quickly led him to the harder ones with the hope that carryover would bring success.

We ourselves experienced difficulty in producing certain consonants, such as /k/, when we used the artificial larynx, or when we tried to demonstrate our own esophageal speech sounds. We began to understand the source of these problems as the researches of the last two decades were reported at conventions and in the literature. We learned among other things that removal of the larynx was responsible for numerous changes in the dynamics of articulation. The anatomical changes caused by removal of the larynx necessitated the use of the PE segment as the source for phonation of voiced sounds. The less refined and weaker vibratory action at the mouth of the PE segment, the neoglottis, might be expected to make the vowels less intelligible. However, the researches of J.O. Anderson; Dicarlo *et al.; and* Hyman showed that vowels are usually heard more distinctively than consonants.*

The lack of firm pulmonary support and the triple duty of the oral and pharyngeal cavities as sites of compression, injection and modification complicates the production of consonants. Consequently final and voiceless consonants and fricatives were found by the above researchers to be the least intelligible of all speech sounds. These errors were especially noticeable in the speech of poor speakers as compared with that of good speakers. The difference between the vowels and consonants in laryngectomees' speech is understandable when we realize that the inherent characteristic spectra of vowels give them the highest intelligibility. This difference remains even in the speech of laryngectomees when the powerful driving force of laryngeal air is replaced by the much weaker

---

* In addition to the researches just mentioned, the reader may obtain a wealth of information from the discussions of Snidecor 1968, and Diedrich and Youngstrom, who have summarized and ably interpreted the significance of research in this new field.

force of esophageal air. This loss also prevents the speaker from sustaining his air support to the production of the final consonant of a phrase or sentence (Fletcher).

Removal of the larynx also necessitates an alteration of the action of the soft palate during articulation of the consonants. It must be raised against the nasopharyngeal port even for the production of nasal sounds, and the lips are closed firmly, in order to create an airtight cavity for compression and injection. The lips, cheeks and tongue are first used to compress and inject the air and then are used for articulating vowels and consonants. When plosive sounds are produced, the articulators may make an additional contribution by injecting some of the air into the esophagus (Damsté; Diedrich and Youngstrom; Moolenaar-Bijl 1953b).

Additional evidence of altered articulation is the observation by Diedrich and Youngstrom that the articulators varied in the production of consonants and vowels when different artificial appliances were used, or when different pharyngeal speakers were heard. Because the tongue has a dual role, first, in compressing and injecting air and then, immediately thereafter, in modifying the ejected air, its contacts and positions during movements are of shorter duration than in normal speech (Diedrich and Youngstrom).

Finally, the unique action of the plosive consonants enables the laryngectomee to use fewer air intakes and to speak longer with a plosive-filled sentence than with a sentence that has few or no plosives. Likewise, the air-splitting nature of the sound /s/ permits fusion of the injection of air with the production of the consonant (Diedrich and Youngstrom).

The person who believes that he can teach esophageal speech simply by showing the laryngectomee how to produce vowels (esophageal sounds) will and should change his mind after he reads the material that has appeared in this text up to this point. If teaching esophageal speech were as easy as such persons have believed, this text would not have been written.

ESOPHAGEAL SPEECH

Air Intake

Three methods of air intake have been mentioned in the literature: swallowing, injection and inhalation (Damsté; Darley 1963; Diedrich and Youngstrom; Froeschels; Hodson and Oswald; McCall; Moolenaar-Bijl 1953a; Moore and Koepp-Baker; Schlosshauer and Möckel; Snidecor; Stetson). The latest research and systematic comparisons of early methods with more recent information have verified some assumptions and have refuted others which were made without verification by direct observation of the physiological action (Damsté; Diedrich and Youngstrom; Snidecor 1968). Recent cinefluorographic studies and spot x-rays have been taken sequentially and simultaneously of the actions and positions of different parts of the speech mechanism during the development of air pressures and the production of vowels and consonants. These views have, for the first time, allowed speech pathologists accurate, direct observation and a much clearer understanding of the different methods by which laryngectomees utilize nonpulmonary air for producing esophageal speech sounds.

Although swallowing (deglutition), inhalation and injection have been the most commonly listed methods of air intake (Diedrich and Youngstrom) or air-charge (Snidecor), cinefluorographic studies show that practically all laryngectomees employ injection or inhalation or both. Twenty of Diedrich's patients were seen to use injection and seven to use inhalation.* Among Damsté's patients, twenty-three used injection and one inhaled air. Isshiki and Snidecor wrote: "Most of the recent investigators appear to refute swallowing per se as a method of air intake in esophageal speech."

Injection

The only air that is immediately available for injection into the esophagus (and for inhalation) is within the mouth and pharyngeal cavities. Before the laryngectomee speaks, he can be seen to make a simple movement of the lips, a movement of the muscles under the chin or a tensing of the cheeks (Moolenaar-Bijl 1953b). Any or all of these actions will help to move air from the front of the mouth to the pharnyx and from there into the esophagus, provided the segment relaxes its sphincterlike opening.

A cinefluorographic side view of this action shows what happens inside the mouth and pharynx during injection. An experienced talker may readily move air into the esophagus by a simple lip action, which may or may not be assisted by compression of the cheeks, or by a "mere flick of the tongue" Damsté 1958). Beginners may squeeze the lips and cheeks several times to move the air. "Slight flick of the tongue" means that an efficient speaker need only lift his tongue slightly to move air; however, a beginner must make a more deliberate effort, first by raising his tongue tip against the alveolar ridge, as in making a /t/, and second, by rocking the rest of the tongue against the hard palate. At the same time, the very essential closure of the soft palate is made to seal off the nasopharyngeal cavity. With the lips closed and the tongue rocking back-

* The following authors' works should give the reader a rather complex history of air intake theories: Damsté, Diedrich and Youngstrom; M.C.L. Greene: Luchsinger and Arnold; Snidecor 1968.

ward, the air is moved into the only opening available, the neoglottis. This deliberate, more complete action of the tongue was named the *glossal press* by Damsté (1959) and Moolenaar-Bijl (1953b) (see also van den Berg *et al.*). It has been regarded by Diedrich and Youngstrom as an act of injection, as revealed by their cinefluorographic studies.

The speaker can force all or most of the air from the mouth and pharynx by a more complete action of the tongue, that is, by continuing the upward and backward thrust to make contact with the posterior wall of the pharynx, which moves slightly forward to meet it. (Not all the air should be expelled from the oral-pharyngeal cavities; otherwise none will be available for the consonant (Diedrich and Youngstrom). This is called the *glosspharyngeal press.* A motion picture view of these two actions, taken while a person is talking, shows that the rapid up and down and backward movement of the tongue is a pistonlike action (Darley 1963; Sawkins; Snidecor). Schilling and Binder, as early as 1927, and others described the action as "pumping action" (Baker; Bateman *et al.*; Marland; Damsté; Moore; Moore and Koepp-Baker; Stetson). The pumping action may vary from light, easy and slightly incomplete to forceful and complete injections. The variations may change with the demands of the speaker for carrying on a light conversation or speaking forcefully and loudly. Fluent speakers generally appear to talk with ease and without exaggerated movements connected with in and out movements of air. These are the ones who may speak with the simple lip movements and slight flicks of the tongue mentioned above.

Plosives as Aids to Injection. An inhalation or injection of air ordinarily must precede every esophageal sound made from a position of rest (Diedrich and Youngstrom). However, during the speaking of a syllable that contains a plosive consonant such as the /p/ in *pah,* part of the air that is compressed enters the esophagus. This is an important addition to the air supply because it permits a longer usage of esophageal air for succeeding sounds and gives more fluency to speech. The sounds that have this air-splitting feature are /p/, /t/, /k/, /tʃ/ (*ch*), /ʃ/ (*sh*) and /s/ (van den Berg *et al.*; Damsté 1959; Diedrich and Youngstrom).

It would appear that if every syllable were to begin with a plosive sound, talking would be much easier. In fact, Moolenaar-Bijl (1953a, 1953b) has suggested that a not quite perceptible (audible) production of any voiceless plosive may be sufficient to inject air into the esophagus to initiate speech. This dynamic arrangement points to the importance of initiating the first esophageal sounds through the use of plosives. We have taken advantage of this phenomenon by warning our patients that they always can get started talking by thinking of or saying /p/.

An additional and very valuable advantage stems from the peculiar ac-

tion of voiceless plosive sounds. If the syllable *pah* is repeated rapidly
in a series, it can be repeated with a longer duration than can the vowel
/a/ alone, the air supply of which diminishes rapidly (Berlin 1963a;
Damsté; Diedrich and Youngstrom; Morrison; Snidecor 1968). Likewise,
words, phrases and sentences that are weighted with voiceless plosive
consonants will be more easily pronounced than words and sentences that
have no plosive sounds. The air-splitting phenomenon of /s/ is different
from the plosive consonants in timing, in that it occurs simultaneously
with its production. The air from the hypopharynx is injected into the
esophagus at the same moment that the sound is produced by compressing
air in the oral cavity. Diedrich and Youngstrom's description of this action
is quite clear:

> A true "fusion" (Stetson) of the consonant and air intake is found when injection
> of air and production of a voiceless sibilant occur simultaneously. Whereas
> in plosive air injection, a sequential unfolding of events occurs, i.e., air injection
> is first and then explosion of the consonant occurs.

TONGUE-LOCK AS AN AID. McClear's (1969) method of injecting air is
designed specifically to train the patient consciously to do two things.
First, he places the tongue tip against the alveolar ridge (upper gum line)
and, "locking" (holding) it there, makes a swallow. Essentially this means
that he rocks the back of the tongue against the palate to compress and
move air back into the pharynx and thence into the esophagus. The patient must consciously learn to perform these movements in order to train
his muscles to develop a new automatic action. He is also directed to
keep his lips parted slightly. This would appear to add to the difficulty
of obtaining compression, but no air leaks from behind the tongue, which
seals off the posterior oral and pharyngeal air. It also helps to teach the
patient to concentrate on the tongue action.

McClear insists that the swallow is not an act of deglutition; rather it
is only the first part of the swallowing act. Van den Berg *et al.* describe it
as follows:

> This scene, as well as following scenes, shows that the injection phenomenon
> starts in just the same way as the first act of swallowing. The esophageal
> sphincter relaxes or yields when the pharyngeal pressure is high enough, and
> the esophagus is loaded. The subsequent phases of swallowing, however, be-
> ginning with the propulsive wave in the oesophagus, towards the stomach and
> the yielding of the cardia, are not initiated; the air remains in the oesophagus
> and can be used for voice production, the oesophagus behaving more or less
> passively.

This injection is the same glossal press we have discussed above, but
McClear trains the patient to do it consciously by emphasizing tongue-
lock and swallowing.

McClear also takes advantage of the air-splitting propulsive action of /s/ and the injecting action of the voiceless plosive consonant to perform a very effective injection of air into the esophagus:

> Say the letter "T" as whispered in the word "Tea." Say the letters "SSSSSS" as whispered in the word "See" or sound like a steam radiator; hiss the villain. Again say the letter "T" as whispered in the word "Tea." This mark is the sign of the tongue lock and it means that you should swallow. Practice this several times to get the feel of the motion of the tongue.

McClear also uses the blends /st/, /sp/ and /sk/ as starters or aids to injection. By using these blends, he has arranged a triple injection in this instruction. He really did not need to ask the patient to "swallow," that is, to use the tongue-lock and swallow. He already had two good injecting actions available, one in the plosive action of /t/ and the other in the impulsion of air by the air-splitting process of /s/. The combination of /st/ thus might have been enough to produce the word *stop* without the tongue-lock injection action.* Adding this third action of tongue-lock injection, he gets a highly explosive response from the esophagus. This would appear, then, to be one of the most effective methods of initiating esophageal sounds. Hence, many teachers use the plosive-pumping technique.

In clinical practice, we had been struggling to initiate an esophageal sound in one patient, and finally suggested that he say *stop*. The word came forth at once, clearly, on the first attempt. Another speech clinician had been working on a patient for three sessions but had had no success with injection or inhalation. He requested us to help out. In five minutes, the man was saying *stop it, speak up, skip it, etc.* This demonstrates vividly the importance of using plosives in initiating esophageal speech sounds, and of being eclectic in trying different methods and materials when one method does not work.

Inhalation

The outstanding difference between injection and direct inhalation of air for use in esophageal speech is the aerodynamic situation in the mouth and throat. Injection generally requires a tight oral-pharyngeal chamber made so by closed lips and closed soft palate. This permits the air within to be compressed and injected into the esophagus, which is the only place it can go (Diedrich and Youngstrom; Moore 1957). Inhalation is done with an open oral-pharyngeal chamber, made so by parted lips and a soft palate more or less open or less tightly approximated than for injection.

---

* Diedrich and Youngstrom, on page 100 of their book, would require injection for the vowel from the rest position for /t/, whereas /sta/ would furnish two impulsions of air.

Furthermore, the tongue is active in injection, which takes the form of a glossal press or glossopharyngeal press, whereas in inhalation the tongue lies in a flat, relaxed position of quite, nearly "motionless activity" (Diedrich and Youngstrom). No swallowing or pumping action is seen during inhalation of air into the esophagus, whereas some authorities state that the action of the tongue in injection resembles the first phase of swallowing (van den Berg *et al.;* Damsté; Schlosshauer and Möckel; Snidecor 1968).

During injection, air enters the esophagus, which may be forced open by a higher pressure within the hypopharynx, as a result of tongue compression, or by a relearned pattern of voluntary relaxation of the neoglottis (Damsté; Snidecor 1968). However, during inhalation, the neoglottis is open. Air enters the esophagus because of the negative pressure (partial vacuum) that is created by the descent of the diaphragm and the expansion of the thorax (Brodnitz; Damsté; M.C.L. Greene; Levin 1962). Since the trachea and the esophagus are positioned side by side, the negative pressure of the thorax alters the pressure in the adjoining esophagus. The air then rushes from the mouth and throat into the open esophagus (Damsté). The speaker feels this as a sensation of sucking in air, as we all do with breathing. He naturally will believe that the inhalation method is the most natural and the easiest way of moving air into the esophagus.

The "Modified Swallow" (Diedrich and Youngstrom)

Many speech clinicians have used the term *swallow* as part of their instructions to take in air for producing esophageal sounds (Gardner 1951, 1964; Laguaite and Waldrop; Levin 1940, 1952; Lindsay *et al.;* Martin 1963; McCall; Morrison). For example, instructions might be (a) open mouth, (b) close mouth, (c) swallow and (d) say *ah* (Doehler; Waldrop and Gould). Although many of the authors wrote in earlier years on the successful use of swallowing, as late as 1963 Martin advocated the swallow-belch as the only technique for moving air in and out of the esophagus for speech.

GASTRIC AIRBALL. Because the esophagus is part of the speech mechanism of a laryngectomee, the word *swallow*, used in teaching esophageal speech, was believed to be equivalent to a command to perform the act of deglutition. This opinion was fortified by the belief that the gastric airball became enlarged during air deglutition and decreased in size after phonation (Luchsinger and Arnold; Morrison 1941). Beck; Cojazzi; van Gilse; and Luchsinger and Arnold proved that the airball in the stomach did not change its size before, during or after esophageal phonation.

PERISTALSIS. When barium is swallowed, it is quickly passed into the esophagus by peristaltic movement and thence through the cardiac sphincter into the stomach. In order to determine how different the swallow is from injection for esophageal speech, Damsté formed into a loop the film strip that showed the true act of swallowing so that he could observe repeatedly the total action. He did the same with injection. In summarizing his observations, he stated that during air injection, the peristaltic movements do not occur, the cardiac sphincter does not open and the air remains in the esophagus for expulsion for speech.*

REFLEX AND VOLUNTARY OPENING OF THE NEOGLOTTIS. Because the esophagus in normal speakers was automatically and unconsciously opened during deglutition in reflex response to a chain of stimuli from the pharyngeal surfaces (Bateman; Damsté), the early investigators believed that the esophagus would be opened in a similar manner during the act of taking in air for esophageal speech. This has been found not to be true. The swallowing (peristaltic) stimuli and peristaltic movements initiated in the pharynx by foods are not present in air injection and hence the esophagus does not receive the serial stimuli which would open the neoglottis (van den Berg *et al.*; Negus). Since the esophagus is not opened reflexly among laryngectomees during speech (being normally closed), it is necessary for the laryngectomee to learn voluntarily to open the neoglottis (Damsté; Diedrich and Youngstrom). However, as we have already discussed in this chapter, the tonicity of the neoglottis is often reduced from surgical procedures.

FIRST STAGE OF SWALLOWING. Some investigators have remarked that the process of injecting air into the esophagus resembles somewhat the first stage of swallowing (Berlin 1964; Damsté; Moolenaar-Bijl; Snidecor). They say that the back of the tongue is lifted, while forcing air into the pharynx, in the same manner in which the tongue forces food from the oral cavity. Diedrich and Youngstrom's meticulous cinefluorographic studies of movements of the speech mechanisms of experienced speakers showed that the injection of air in the form of a pumping action was different from swallowing. For example, in the glossopharyngeal action for swallowing food, the tongue contacted the posterior portion of the pharyngeal wall in order to "strip" the food away and to force it downward. During the glossopharyngeal press for injecting air, the back of the tongue only momentarily "bumped" the posterior wall of the pharynx. Diedrich and Youngstrom therefore recommended:

> It is probably not helpful to describe the process of air intake as one of deglutition. In teaching esophageal speech, the subject must learn something different than "swallow the air" in order to be successful at air intake.

For this reason, they called the injection process a "modified swallow."

* Read page 289 of Luchsinger and Arnold and page 104 of Diedrich and Youngstrom for historical narratives of the investigations of gastric movements related to postlaryngectomy speech.

DIFFERENCES IN PALATAL ACTION. The altered action of the palate mentioned above also facilitates the development of pressure in the oral-
pharyngeal cavity. In swallowing, the soft palate is raised and loosely
approximated to the nasal pharyngeal opening. However, during esophageal speech, the soft palate is raised tightly against the opening (van den
Berg *et al.*; Diedrich and Youngstrom). This sealing action occurs even
when the speaker produces nasal sounds. However, the tight closure may
later be slackened somewhat when the speaker develops skill in compressing and injecting (Diedrich and Youngstrom).

DIFFERENCES IN THE SPEED OF SWALLOWING. Another difference between
the swallowing actions for food and for the injection of air is the change
in the speed of swallowing. Motta *et al.* quoted Janker and Schwab as observing that the food bolus moved more slowly through the pharynx of
the laryngectomee than in normal persons. Janowski *et al.* more specifically
observed that some of the barium that remained in the hypopharynx of a
laryngectomee after one swallow was removed by subsequent swallows.
While confirming this, Diedrich and Youngstrom went farther by measuring the speed of swallowing of normal and laryngectomized persons. The
time taken from the first initiation of movement for the bolus to go from
a position of rest to the point where it exits from the PE segment was
0.50 second for normals and 1.00 second for laryngectomees (Diedrich
and Youngstrom). It was also found that one-third of the patients thus
measured delayed the normal pattern of closing off the soft palate simultaneously with entry of the bolus into the esophagus. Thus, even in the
process of eating, the action of swallowing of laryngectomees is modified.
Over one-third of Diedrich and Youngstrom's patients surveyed reported
that swallowing was more difficult; one-third took longer to eat; almost
60 per cent took smaller swallows and chewed their food better (before
swallowing). These points led Diedrich and Youngstrom to conclude that
the pattern of deglutition could not be used for rapid esophageal speech.

IMPLICATIONS FOR THOSE WHO SWALLOW. After all of this discussion in
proving that air injection is different from food swallowing, we still face
a problem with swallowers. Damsté says that a patient may start with
swallowing, but will eventually discover by himself the knack of injection.
Moolenaar-Bijl states, "After the new speech process has become automatized, however (and this may be very soon), it is no more air swallowing
but sucking or aspirating" (Moolenaar-Bijl 1951).

It is understandable for patients to use deglutition if their teachers use
the word *swallow* in their instructions. We have seen patients who had
been taught that way who could only use one syllable for each air-charge.
They often took five seconds to swallow air, meanwhile endeavoring to
collect some saliva. Some kept lozenges handy so that they could obtain

a swallow stimulus. When they got the sound it came forth with a loud burst. The speech clinician may have been at fault because he did not explain that the air-charge was a "modified swallow." Even at that the teacher or his patients may not have understood that injection was something different from swallowing (Damsté; Diedrich and Youngstrom) and that they had to learn an entirely different muscular pattern (van den Berg and Moolenaar-Bijl). (Johnson found that using the word *swallow* caused his patients to use muscles that were associated with swallowing.)

CHANGING THE SWALLOW PATTERN. We believe with others (Snidecor) that the term *swallow* should be replaced by *pump, inject* or *charge* (Diedrich and Youngstrom). We can do two things. First, we can avoid giving the wrong impression by using voiceless plosives or inhalation to initiate air intake, or, if the patient develops a swallow pattern, we can quickly change it by using plosives for injection or by using inhalation, in which the tongue must be kept flat. Finally, working toward getting air in fast and out fast (Berlin 1963b; Snidecor), the speech clinician can train the patient to alter the slow swallow into one of rapid injection. Since he cannot swallow fast, he is forced to change his pattern to something else. Thus, those few beginners who do swallow air will quickly learn a more effcient method (Damsté).

It behooves us always to remain eclectic in our technique. This means that we can resort to mimicking the swallow if no other methods succeed. And our contemporaries all admit that with some difficult cases, they have had to resort to sips and swallows of liquids, even with carbonated water added, to establish a kinesthetic image of what they wanted.

AEROPHAGIA. A final point that has not been discussed by any investigators other than Luchsinger and Arnold is aerophagia. A patient who has this habit has already learned to inject air into the esophagus. Moreover, since he is experienced in producing an immediate belch after injection, as we have also observed among some of our functionally dysphonic patients, he has merged the two actions into an almost simultaneous "in and out" action. Since this is the goal we seek for all laryngectomees (Snidecor), we can conclude that laryngectomized aerophagics have modified their swallowing pattern even before they have had instruction in esophageal speech.

Air Expulsion

After air has been injected into the subneoglottal air chamber (esophagus), it must be moved out (expelled) under a pressure that will set into vibration the walls of the forward portion of the PE segment (neoglottis), the mouth of which merges with the hypopharynx. The vibrating air is then moved through the oral-pharyngeal cavity for modification into vowels and voiced consonants.

Van den Berg *et al.* stressed the importance of keeping the pressure of air constant within the esophagus while the laryngectomee phonates. Isshiki and Snidecor showed that most of the outward flow of air from the esophagus or oral-pharyngeal cavity occurred during the exhalatory phase of respiration (synchrony), regardless of the method of air intake. It therefore is logical to believe that there is a relationship between exhalation and phonation (Diedrich and Youngstrom; M.C.L. Greene; Luchsinger and Arnold; Robe *et al.* 1956c). In fact, Snidecor states that exhalation of lung air facilitates the expulsion of air from the esophagus. The most effective proof of this is to determine how speakers meet the demand for more pressure that is necessary for loud speech. A dramatic narration by Snidecor revealed one way in which this was accomplished. The speaker simply inhaled more deeply and spoke loudly with his esophageal voice. Likewise, the need for more air for speaking a longer phrase usually is preceded by a deeper inspiration of lung air. Furthermore, if a person exhausts his esophageal air before he finishes a phrase, he will try futilely to breathe out harder (blow air from the stoma) to support the final sound. This shows that some kind of correlating action between exhalation and phonation must be present during periods of loud or extended duration of speech.

A clue to the source of the pressure that occurs within the thorax as a result of respiration is obtained from observing external application of pressure on the esophagus. Needing sufficient pressure to expel air, some speakers will press a finger on the neck where it is possible to feel the swallowing of liquid or passing of air downward. In fact, this is practiced regularly by teachers in initiating esophageal speech among difficult cases. Speech clinicians frequently fasten a small sponge to a tape which is tied behind the neck (McClear 1959). The tape holds the sponge, placed in front against the neck in order to narrow the airway. We also have observed laryngectomees pressing their hands against their chest while they talked. When we asked them to speak without using the hand pressure, either they had difficulty starting speech or their voice was weakened.

The last two examples of applied pressure give us a clue to the nature of the mechanism that creates and maintains pressure during phonation. Pressure must be developed within the thoracic cavity in such a manner that it increases the pressure within the esophagus. For this, van den Berg *et al.* believe that two outstanding mechanisms are available:

1. When a person exhales, the pressure that rises within the trachea is transmitted through its walls to the adjoining esophagus. If

the esophagus is already filled from injection, the added pressure from the outside is great enough to produce a louder voice or a longer phrase (Diedrich and Youngstrom; M.C.L. Greene, Levin 1955; Lindsay *et al.*; Seeman 1967).

2. The second important force comes from the elastic quality of the nonmuscular components of the walls of the esophagus. It permits the walls to expand and/or contract in a manner that maintains a constant pressure. This answers the requirement of van den Berg *et al.* that a constantly adjusting pressure is necessary to produce a steady flow of air supply for speech.

Damsté (1958) aptly describes the final action of expulsion:

> If the sphincter of the oesophageal mouth is under good control, the pressure under which the air is pumped into the oesophagus can be used instantaneously for speaking one or two syllables. The pressure is maintained for some time due to the elasticity and the muscle tonus of the oesophageal wall. However, only for a very short time, then the air is carried off by a peristaltic wave. Hence, we see that injection and phonation are not two separate phases but constitute one whole.

The quick in-and-out action described here emphasizes the need for those forces which can act forcefully and almost instantaneously, and can sustain the pressure while the speaker phonates.

Other suggested sources of aid to expulsion have been made:

1. Abdominal support (Diedrich and Youngstrom).

2. Compression from the rise of the diaphragm in exhalation (Snidecor).

3. Retrograde contraction of the esophagus (Schlosshauer and Möckel; Seeman 1967).

4. Active contraction of the voluntary (striated) muscles of the forward end of the esophagus (van den Berg *et al.*).

However, van den Berg *et al.* believe that these factors are minor to the above two basic ones in that they are not needed or are not as important in expelling air from the esophagus. However, they all may make a contribution to the desired sustained pressure during speech. Moreover, practically all of the factors presented above indicate the importance of correlating respiration and phonation in the speech instruction of laryngectomees (DiCarlo *et al.*; Motta *et al.*; Robe *et al.* 1956b; Schlosshauer and Möckel; Stetson 1937a).

PHARYNGEAL SPEECH

Although the patient has the PE segment with its neoglottis for vibratory purposes, he may not produce the usual esophageal sound for one or more reasons. The muscles of the neoglottis may be so highly tonic that they cannot be opened voluntarily. The patient may not comprehend instructions and by chance may approximate surfaces in the pharyngeal area to produce a sound which he thinks is what is wanted. Damsté says that numerous folds, constrictions and stenoses may be sites for approximations to form a pseudoglottis. Martin states that the vibrating surfaces for pharyngeal speech may be at any level from the cricopharyngeal muscle up to the base of the tongue, or at any place where healing of tissues leaves a prominent or roughened surface. Both Morrison and Kallen define the pharyngeal voice as being produced in a pseudoglottis located somewhere in the oro- or hypopharynx with its air chamber below that point. Diedrich and Youngstrom suggest that the pseudoglottis may be formed by the tongue being approximated against the hard and soft palates, tonsillar pillars or posterior pharyngeal wall, with the hypopharynx serving as the air chamber. One of our patients gave an interesting example of pharyngeal voice. He had been referred by a laryngologist because he had acquired a peculiar voice while being taught to swallow air. In an agonizing effort to inject and expel air, the patient jammed his tongue against the junction between the soft and hard palates. Bubbles of saliva sputtered out between the surfaces as he squeezed out a thin, high-pitched sound.* Fortunately, we heard an occasional undertone at a lower pitch which we suspected came from the neoglottis. By using plosive consonants and getting the patient to drop his tongue after injection, we succeeded in obtaining a good esophageal sound.

The extreme case of pharyngeal voice just presented probably is just one of the types of cases described by earlier writers who did not have cinefluorograms for the ultimate in simultaneous observation of speech parts in action during pharyngeal and esophageal speech. This is probably true of the report of Waldrop and Toht, whose sonograms of pharyngeal speech resembled normal speech more than esophageal speech, and whose pharyngeal speech Diedrich and Youngstrom suspected was esophageal speech by injection (glossal press or glossopharyngeal press). Sawkins (1952) protested that air was not swallowed in esophageal speech, as we had first described it (Gardner 1951); rather, it was set in motion by gulping air into the pharynx in this manner:

1. Place the tip of the tongue behind the upper front teeth.
2. Raise the root of the tongue toward the roof of the mouth.
3. Set the air into motion by a pistonlike motion of the tongue,

---

* Perello states that patients who use the pharyngeal voice have a low-intensity speech understandable only to persons nearby. This occurs because the sound is squeezed out and is not supported by esophageal vibrations.

that is, a rise and fall. The air is vibrated between the back of the tongue and the posterior wall of the pharynx.

Sawkins, of course, did not and could not have seen the action within the pharynx or within the subneoglottic chamber, or the vibration of the neoglottic lips. He did not realize that his term *pistonlike movement* was describing quite clearly what is now called *injection by glossopharyngeal press* (Damsté). Sawkins gave another clue to the true nature of the speech pattern when he recommended the use of plosive-laden words to initiate sounds, such as *tip, tight, cot* and *ship.*

Nelson also described what he thought was pharyngeal speech. He varied his method by placing the tongue tip against the lower front teeth. He then forced the air backward by arching the middle of the tongue sharply against the roof of the mouth. When a sharp thump was heard the patient produced a speech sound. Since Diedrich and Youngstrom have seen these actions many times and have identified them (including the thump) as injection by glossal press or glossopharyngeal press, they are convinced that what most people call pharyngeal speech is probably esophageal. If this is true, then pharyngeal speech is to be regarded as quite rare.†

Diedrich and Youngstrom suggest that pharyngeal speech should be described as a modification of esophageal voice. It has also been suggested that pharyngeal speech may occur in the process of training a person to inject air when the patient makes his first adjustment of the tongue and pharynx (Damsté, 1958; Moolenaar-Bijl, 1953b). We have corrected such a problem by explanation, demonstration and practice or by shift of therapy to the use of plosive consonants (M.C.L. Greene).

M.C.L. Greene reported one pharyngeal speech case in which the voice was quacky, harsh and ugly. Diedrich and Youngstrom reported a high-pitched, thin sound which issued from a pseudoglottis that was slightly above the true neoglottis, but the patient still used the esophageal reservoir. Damsté *et al.* have described pharyngeal speech as being high-pitched and weak, with dull, slow scanning speech that cannot be modulated by melodic, dynamic or temporal accentuation. The patient is unable to make an initial vowel because he has no air from the esophagus. There is no intentional belch; frequent interruptions for loading are necessary because of the low capacity of the air chamber. With these descriptions,

---

* M.C.L. Greene mentioned Sawkins as "Miss Oswald's highly accomplished laryngectomized speaker." We recall that Miss Oswald taught inhalation as the method of taking in air (Hodson and Oswald).

† Interesting reading is found in Diedrich and Youngstrom's treatment (page 106 of their book) of the research papers of Micheli-Pellegrini, Ragaglini and Teramo, who sought to prove that the hypopharynx was the vicarious air chamber for pharyngeal speech.

speech clinicians should be able to identify pharyngeal speech and take measures to alter it to esophageal speech.

BUCCAL SPEECH

Friction noises are made when the tongue compresses and squeezes air out of a small chamber created by its approximation with the cheek, alveolar ridge or hard palate. The sound has been called *pseudowhisper* because that is all that can be produced (Malbeck and Schlosshauer). The high-pitched squeaky consonants are not only hard to produce and to sustain, but are most difficult to understand as a medium of communication. *

SPEECH BY THE PULMONARY DERMAL-HYPOPHARYNGEAL AIR LOOP

Recent efforts to restore voice in a laryngectomee through surgical techniques have been reported in the literature (Conley *et al.;* Miller 1967; Snidecor 1968). After Miller observed the technique used by Dr. Ryozo Asai of Japan, he performed three-stage operations on nine patients. The ultimate result was the construction of a dermal tube between the stub or upper end of the trachea and the hypopharyx. The pharyngeal end of the tube bends downward in order to prevent direct entry of liquids. Some patients have to press this area with the finger at the moment liquids are swallowed. The usual stoma is somewhat lower.

The upper end of the dermal tube is narrowed to a diameter of 4 mm. Pulmonary air, being driven through this narrow passage, creates a vibratory action of the walls and serves as the pseudoglottis. Miller asserts that six of his first nine patients who had the three-stage operation have voices that are superior to the voices of esophageal speakers. Snidecor studied a selected group of Asai's patients whom he considered were developing as good speech as had been reported by Miller. If the vocal successes continue to be maintained through this type of surgery, the voices of future laryngectomees will be developed with much less difficulty, especially because the patients will have pulmonary air to support their phonation rather than the weaker esophageal expulsion and the infrapharyngeal-oral compression of the present laryngectomees. We believe, however, that these people will require retraining as does the esophageal speaker or the user of the artificial larynx.

A different approach to retaining use of pulmonary air is being developed by Stanley Taub, M.D. Taking advantage of a pharyngeal fistula in his patient, Dr. Staub connected this opening to the stoma by means of an

---

* See Luchsinger and Arnold for a complete analysis of parabuccal and pharyngeal speech.

aluminum device that basically functions like the L-shaped Western Electric Pneumatic Larynx. One L-end is inserted into the stoma and the other L-end into the pharyngeal fistula. The middle section contains a reed in a vibrating chamber that resonates the air from the lungs and passes it to the pharynx. Dr. Taub prepared the fistular-dermal hypopharyngeal tube so that food could not easily enter the device.

In order to wear and hold the aluminum instrument, the patient wears an absorbent collar that contains holes that match the fistula and stoma openings, into which the two ends of the device are inserted. Worn outside the neck, it is snugly held in place and is not visible when the patient wears a shirt and tie.

The middle chamber is shaped to resonate a sound that resembles the average male voice. Dr. Taub introduced one of his patients to the members of the IAL convention which was held at Buffalo, New York, on July 28, 1970. The patient spoke with a slightly husky, but strong, commanding voice which had some of the quality of the Western Electric instrument. He counted from 1 to 30 on one breath; he had enough air to blow out a match. His pitch range was almost one octave. The articulation was excellent. Some laryngectomees thought the device amazing; others said that they would not want to fuss with the contraption because of the mucus problem. Although the present surgical procedure costs considerable time and money, it appears to be another step in the direction of developing an effective medium of communication for the laryngectomee without having to learn esophageal speech.

THE ARTIFICIAL LARYNX

Numerous appliances have been constructed in the past and in recent years to serve as a substitute larynx for those who cannot talk with residual organs or who prefer to use such instruments.* The ingenuity of laryngologists and physicists has resulted in models which can be kept inside the mouth, inserted into the mouth while in use, placed against the throat or actually embedded in the tissues of the neck. For power, early users pumped air with a bellows or used pulmonary air, and later users have had electrical, electronic and wireless models.

History and Types of Instruments

The artificial larynx is a substitute for the voice that is lost when the larynx is partially obstructed or when it is removed through surgery.

---

* Persons who are interested in the history of the artificial larynx may consult the following writers: Barney; Damsté; Diedrich and Youngstrom; Kallen; Luchsinger and Arnold; Morrison 1931; and Perello 1953.

Whether the patient's neoglottis is functioning normally or abnormally, the artificial larynx may also be substituted for that organ.

The first recorded use of an artificial larynx was by a person who had complete atresia of the larynx. In 1859, the laryngologist Czermak and a scientist, Brucke, devised a reed-type vibrator (Kallen). Air from the stoma activated the vibrator, and its vibrations were transmitted into the mouth. Models were revised and used by laryngectomized patients during the last quarter of the nineteenth century. Instruments were the preferred substitute voice because only rarely was a laryngectomee able to use what later was called esophageal voice. As late as 1950, the artificial larynx was routinely issued by many laryngologists.

The artificial larynx today may be classified according to the source of its energy and the application of this energy to the speech mechanism.* The sources of energy are pneumatic (lung air), electrical, electronic and radionic. The instrument may be applied to the neck, inserted within the mouth while speaking or fixed in the mouth.

The Pneumatic Artificial Larynx

The Western Electric Pneumatic Artificial Larynx, first introduced in 1926, was a double-L-shaped silver tube (Fig. 4). One end was inserted in the opening of the tracheotomy tube or in a flexible rubber gasket that fitted tightly over the stoma. Lung air passed from the stoma into the near end and from there into the middle section, which housed a metal reed. Passing over the reed and thereby vibrating it, the air moved into the other end of the "L," to which was attached a rubber flexible tube that was inserted into the mouth of the patient. An opening in the middle section controlled by the thumb permitted the patient either to breathe through the opening or, if it was closed with the thumb, to direct the air over the reed. Although this instrument is no longer manufactured, the parts for it may be obtained through any local office of the Bell Telephone Company.

The sound was low-pitched and monotonous. Loudness and pitch were increased through lung power, but within the limitations of the reed's motility. Thus, the patient was able to emphasize and inflect to a limited degree. He used it in crowds and noisy places and over telephones.

The pneumatic instrument was truly a "lifesaver" for those who survived laryngectomy. Many were able to communicate at once and to return to their jobs.

---

* The history, development, classification and evaluation of the artificial larynx may be found in Arnold; Diedrich and Youngstrom; Luchsinger and Arnold; Martin 1963; Perello 1953; Snidecor 1968; and Van Riper and Irwin.

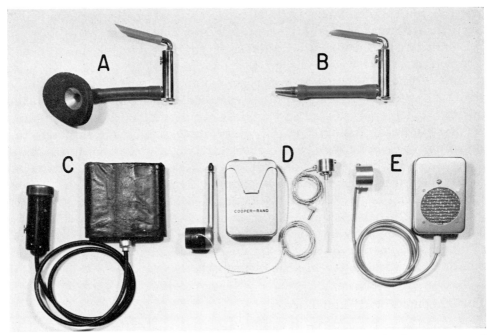

Figure 4. Artificial larynges. *A.* Western Electric Pneumatic Artificial Larynx, reed type: rubber gasket held over stoma, rubber tube held in mouth. *B.* same model, with longer tube inserted in tracheal cannula. *C.* Original model of Aurex Electric Larynx (neck type). *D.* Cooper-Rand Electronic Larynx: transducer is inserted in smoking pipe (left of chassis); transducer is shown on right of chassis with plastic tube to be held in in mouth. *E.* Rand Esophageal Speech Amplifier. (*Courtesy of American Medical Association*)

A member of a Lost Chord Club was supervisor of over 300 maintenance men of a communication system. Although he had understandable speech in close conversation, he found it easier to give his orders over the wires with the instrument in order to insure accuracy. He carried the appliance loosely in his coat pocket where dust and tobacco particles clung to the saliva-moistened mouthpiece that he had to wipe off before inserting into his mouth for talking. He kept an extra metal reed in his pocket as insurance against failure. He maintained in good working order two extra chasses with batteries and connecting wires. One chassis could be used while his wife cleaned the metal and replaced the rubber parts on the spare.

A small, inexpensive, hand-assembled pneumatic model, made in Holland* consists of a flexible plastic cup with an inflated collar, which is pressed tightly against the stoma to receive air from the lungs (Fig. 5). A plastic valve that can be vibrated by lung air is inserted into the base of the cup and connected to a plastic tube that is held in the mouth. The speaker holds the cup over the stoma with one hand and places the tube

* See the Appendix for addresses of manufacturers of the models mentioned here. See also Diedrich and Youngstrom; Snidecor 1968.

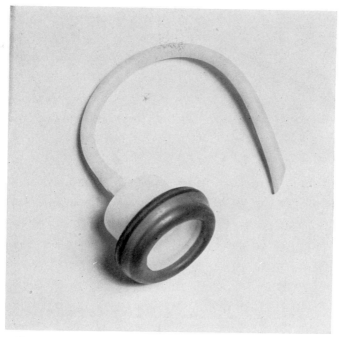

Figure 5. Van Hunen pneumatic larynx model. Flexible head is held closely over the stoma for air pressure; tube is held in mouth. (*Courtesy of W.M. Diedrich and K.A. Youngstrom*)

in his mouth with the other. A home-made version of this model is shown in Figure 6. A Japanese model (Fig. 6), which resembles the old Bell Telephone pneumatic model but is made of plastic valves and tubes, is inexpensive and produces a strong voice. A small piece of rubber dam is fastened over the valve opening to serve as the vibrator. It is easily replaced, and produces a loud voice. A Korean model is an imitation of the Bell Telephone pneumatic larynx. Vibration is produced by inserting a piece of rubber dam between the middle section and the mouthpiece (Fig. 6).

The Electrical Artificial Larynx

The first successful electro-larynx was developed by J. Greene and G. Wright in 1942 (Luchsinger and Arnold), and was sold by the Aurex Corporation, which has developed several models (Fig. 4C). It had a battery-operated vibrator which activated a flat circular diaphragm located at the upper end of a cylindrical container. A large triple-battery container, connected by wires to the base of the cylinder, was carried in the pocket of the user. The diaphragm was held firmly against the side of the neck or in a midline position beneath the chin, wherever it was possible to get the best transmission of sound into the pharynx and mouth. The vibra-

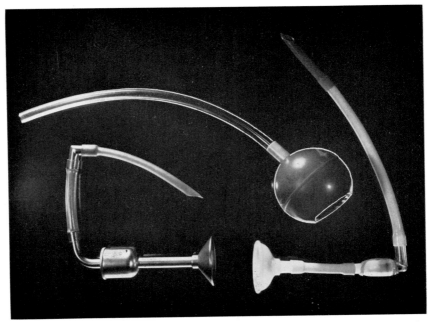

Figure 6. Inexpensive pneumatic models of larynges. *Top:* Homemade type after van Hunen. Ball with open end is held against stoma; tube is held in mouth of speaker. *Left:* Korean all-metal type. Rubber dam is inserted between middle section and neck piece. *Right:* Japanese all-plastic model. Rubber dam is fastened across valve in center. Flexible plastic piece is held over stoma and long tube is held in mouth (Rev. Y. Yamamura).

tions traveling by means of the body tissues were modified into vowels and voiced consonants. The auditor was occasionally distracted when the patient permitted the vibrations to escape into the free air. The electrolarynx has been improved by the Aurex Corporation and by others. Besides improving the quality of the tone and the volume, Aurex created a small, compact, battery-contained cylinder with the vibrating disc on one end as in the original model (Fig. 7). This model has been very popular because of its small size and ease of maintenance, as has the Kett, Mark III.

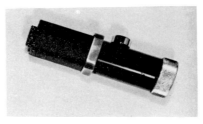

Figure 7. Revised Aurex artificial larynx with self-contained battery and vibrator. Kett Mark III is somewhat similar. (*Courtesy of W.M. Diedrich and K.A. Youngstrom*)

Electronic Models

THROAT TYPE. A recent variation of the throat vibrator appliance is the Bell Telephone Electronic Artificial Larynx (Fig. 8), which is obtainable at the local commercial departments of the Bell Telephone Company. Its battery-contained cylinder is shaped and tapered for the hand at one end and is enlarged at the other end to hold a round plastic diaphragm which lies on

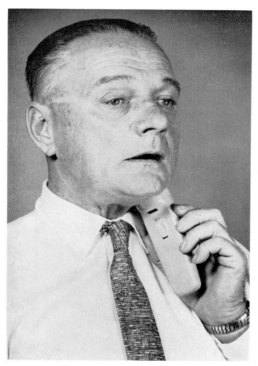

Figure 8. Laryngectomee demonstrating Bell Telephone Electronic Artificial Larynx (neck type). (*Courtesy of American Medical Association*)

a 60-degree plane from the longitudinal axis. The altered angle permits an easier placement of the diaphragm against the neck. A knob-type switch controls a pitch-intensity range which enables the speaker to vary his speech for inflection, emphasis and stress, and which thereby gives him a more natural and less monotonous speech than the older models. The range is long enough to permit someone to sing "America" by depressing the switch control knob at various levels. Servicing the model seems to be minimal, and the two 3.4-volt batteries are quickly installed. Two models are available, the higher-pitched one giving the female a more feminine voice.

TUBE-IN-THE-MOUTH TYPE. The Cooper-Rand Electronic Larynx (Fig. 4D) is an electronic self-powered pulse generator housed in a flat box about the size of a cigarette package. Connected to the chassis by fine wires is a small hand-held transducer which resembles a hearing aid receiver. Pressure on its tiny switch button activates the generation of vibrations which are transmitted through a plastic tube leading from the transducer to the mouth. The end of the tube must be held to one side of the tongue in order to permit the tongue free movement. The speaker also must avoid plugging the open end of the tube, which happens when it touches the surfaces of the tongue or cheek. Controls on the box are used to modify vibrations for varying intensities and pitches. These allow greater flexibility and reduce monotony. One of our club members, a pipe salesman, inserted his transducer into the bowl of his pipe. His sales improved markedly as he was known as the man who talked through his pipe. He used the same idea as Ticchioni of Milan, Italy, who originated the pipe idea for his electronic artificial larynx.

IN-THE-MOUTH TYPE. The English model by Tait (Snidecor 1968) has a miniature diaphragm that is encased in a plastic dental prosthesis. The vibrations are activated from a chassis that is carried in the pocket. It is necessary for the wearer to keep in his mouth a wire that connects the prosthesis with the chassis. H.K. Cooper, DDS., has also prepared a similar prosthetic dental plate. (See page 145 of Diedrich and Youngstrom.)

The Radionic Artificial Larynx

J.H. Pichler, of Vienna, Austria, has been developing a wireless prosthetic device that consists of a tiny speaker embedded in a denture. Vibrations are activated by the speech-respiratory reflex, the sound being transmitted from an induction loop that is worn around the neck. Pichler claims that the appliance produces undistorted consonants.

Physiological Bases of Speech with the Artificial Larynx

The laryngectomee who speaks with an artificial larynx has one advantage over the esophageal speaker. He need not perform as much muscular activity to communicate as does the esophageal speaker. It is not necessary for his tongue to inject the oral-pharyngeal air into the esophagus for voice, and then in turn to quickly articulate for consonants. The appliance furnishes the vibrations for the voice. However, there is no airflow from the trachea and larynx; both types of speakers must use the tongue to compress the air within the oral-pharyngeal cavities and then modify it for the plosive and sibilant consonants.*

Likewise, the tongue must compress intraoral-pharyngeal air for the production of the plosive and sibilant components of consonants (/b/, /d/, /z/, etc.) that are voiced either by the injection-expulsion process or by the artificial larynx. Transmitting or inducing vibrations within the oral-pharyngeal cavities for modification varies not only between the method used in esophageal speech and the one used with appliances but also between the methods of the different appliances (Diedrich and Youngstrom). In esophageal speech, the oral-pharyngeal air injected into the esophagus is immediately set into vibration as it is expelled, and is transmitted upward and forward into the oral-pharyngeal cavities for the shaping of the vowel or voiced consonant. In speech with the electro-larynx, the vibrating diaphragm is applied externally to the neck so that the vibrations enter through the skin into the hypopharynx and mouth. In the tube-in-the mouth type, the vibrations are piped into the mouth, that is, they are delivered in the front of the mouth instead of from the back and then forward. In the in-the-mouth type; vibrations originate within the mouth at the level of the teeth.

With all of this information, we can understand why Diedrich and Youngstrom's cinefluoroscopic study of a patient showed that the patient used three slightly different patterns of tongue action when he spoke, respectively, with esophageal speech, with the Cooper-Rand tube-in-the-mouth larynx and with the Aurex throat-type of appliance.

An outstanding example of consonants whose production cannot be aided by the use of an artificial larynx is the sound /k/. The normal speaker lifts the tongue against the palate to build up pressure of the air streaming from the larynx, then suddenly drops the tongue to release the compressed air. The esophageal speaker cannot produce the /k/ easily because no air pressure is furnished by the larynx. Consequently, the tongue must trap and compress air to develop pressure in the pharynx before it can be released forward. A similar procedure must be used to produce all consonants, with the exception of their voiced components.

The artificial larynx which presents the vibration through a tube inserted into the mouth appears to have two weaknesses (Diedrich and Youngstrom; Snidecor). By holding the tube between the lips, the airtight seal for compression is broken. Likewise, the sound may be completely stopped if the tongue occludes the inward end. In our own use of such an appliance, we soon learned to avoid obstruction of the sound and as-

---

* Diedrich and Youngstrom believe that some air may come from the neoglottis to be used for consonant production, provided it does not vibrate and is eased out slowly.

sumed that laryngectomees would quickly do likewise. The loss of the seal need not be too much of a problem because some teachers of esophageal speech request the patient to open the lips purposely, or even to bite a pencil, in order to force him to make a tight tongue-palate seal. We have found this a valuable technique in teaching esophageal speech.

Another common characteristic of the artificial larynx is the constant monotonous drone of the vibrator. However, the more recent appliances, such as the Bell throat type, permit flexibility of pitch and intensity (loudness) by simply pressing the button farther or releasing pressure. An experienced user can become quite adept in manipulating the switch to obtain flexibility and approach normalcy of speech.

Another common problem is the need for manipulating the switch to match pauses between phrases and for breathing. This, too, has been developed to a fine skill by experienced users. One person who talks probably at the rate of 300 words a minute has acquired rapid manipulation of the switch to produce a rather natural type of conversation. Speech clinicians should explain to users of the artificial larynx that they should pay special attention to this detail. As a matter of fact, this technique should be systemically drilled into them.

Advantages and Disadvantages of the Artificial Larynx

Table I contains statements about the advantages and disadvantages of using the artificial larynx. It is interesting that the arguments gleaned from the literature supporting one viewpoint are opposed by similar arguments supporting the other side. This inconsistency is shown also in the results of research that has been done on loudness, intelligibility and acceptability (Crouse; DiCarlo *et al.*; Hyman; McCroskey and Mulligan; Shames *et al.*). Diedrich and Youngstrom summarize the research studies as follows:

> Certainly, the differences found between the esophageal speakers and users of the artificial larynx are not clearcut. Based on listener judgments of intelligibility, the research does not warrant the strongly biased opinion of some clinicians that esophageal speech is naturally superior to the artificial larynx. . . . If we look at the communication disorder of the patient and not at "best methods of talking," we might be able to formulate some different views about the tools and methods which are available to serve him. . . . It is proposed that the dichotomy between esophageal speech and the artificial larynx also be abandoned, since we do not exist in an either-or world, but within a continuum of alternatives.

Further remarks concerning the research are that it was done with what might be called two perfect systems of communication, the speakers

TABLE I
ADVANTAGES AND DISADVANTAGES OF ARTIFICIAL LARYNX*

Advantages	*Disadvantages*
1. Can always talk with less risk of failing to acquire esophageal speech.	26. No patients or only "a few" are satisfied with it; most abandon it after learning esophageal speech.
2. Permits prompt speech at any time.	27. All are anxious to discard it, even though successful speakers with it.
3. Is easily understood over telephone.	28. If patient uses instrument and learns to talk with it, he will be reluctant to give it up, or will not take time or trouble to learn esophageal speech.
4. Useful at times, even when one uses esophageal speech, e.g., in noise, with weak voice, in urgent situations, under strained conditions and when patient has a cold.	29. It is a constant reminder of a disability.
5. Useful when patient has physical limitations.	30. It points to a social stigma.
6. Useful when patient fails to learn esophageal speech.	31. It attracts unwanted attention and curiosity because it is conspicuous both visually and aurally (it is noisy).
7. Gives early communication by patient to relatives, friends, workers, over telephone.	32. Is bulky and awkward to handle.
8. Useful for early return to work with later success in learning esophageal speech.	33. Is not identified with the speaker's personality as is "natural" esophageal speech.
9. Necessary for early return to work to ease finances, protect own business, retain job.	34. Is less apt to give physical and psychological benefits than is esophageal speech.
10. Prevents discomfort of auditors who would be upset over poor esophageal speech or silence.	35. Is a distraction to auditor and speaker.
11. Prevents fatigue when conditions demand loud speech or extensive talking.	36. Requires use of one hand.

12. Learning to speak with an appliance is achieved
  a. More easily than in esophageal speech.
  b. In a very short time (quicker than esophageal speech).
  c. With less muscular effort.
	37. Maintenance is expensive; hard to clean.
	38. Breakdown or loss is a hazard at critical moments; makes patient helpless.
	39. Is the easiest way out for surgeon and patient.

13. Is more easily understood than esophageal speech.	40. Is not a good substitute for speech.
14. Is better than writing, which delays communication and takes 25 per cent more time.	41. Sound of instrument does not resemble natural human speech.
15. Is better than whispering.	42. Is less dependable than esophageal speech.
16. Is free of grimaces, stoma noise, burps.	43. Speech is no better than "fair" esophageal speech.
17. Voice has more uniform vocal quality; is less raucous; is more acceptable.	44. Speech is unnatural, raucous, metallic, monotonous, etc.
18. Volume is better in noise than with esophageal speech.	45. Lacks volume.
19. Has good intelligibility.	46. Instrument noises reduce intelligibility.
20. Permits communication with instructor during early period of instruction.	47. Speech is distorted, machinelike.
21. Patients who use an artificial larynx acquire esophageal speech well in a shorter time than those who begin with esophageal speech.	48. Is awkward to use for casual remarks because one is not quickly available.
22. Vowels and consonant-vowel syllables have a shorter duration than in esophageal speech.	49. Is a sign of defeat.
23. Sounds in speech with the artificial larynx are not as seriously altered as in esophageal speech.	50. Patient does not think he is doing the talking.
24. Artificial larynx is something one can always fall back on.	
25. Prevents depression by giving the patient early use of artificial larynx, i.e., communication.	

* The statements in this table were taken from the following authors. They do not in all cases reflect the authors' opinions. In many instances the authors merely indicated or listed the advantages and disadvantages offered by users and/or by other authors: Bangs *et al.*; Brodnitz; Damsté 1958; Damsté *et al.* 1956; Diedrich; Equen; M.C.L. Greene; Heaver *et al.*; Howie; Kallen; Lauder; Levin 1940, 1952, 1955; Long; Luchsinger and Arnold; Martin 1963; Miller; Morrison; Orton; Pitkin; Shanks; Snidecor; Van Riper and Irwin; West *et al.* Item 48 is a common complaint among some users of the artificial larynx and among observers of the users' problems.

being superior in their communication. However, if the entire group of speakers, poor and good, were used, there would be no argument about the superiority of esophageal speech over the speech obtainable from the artificial larynx. Likewise, a glance at the nature of the arguments shows that the criticisms against the artificial larynx are concerned more with the psychological problems that might be associated with the use of an instrument, whereas the arguments in favor of the instrument are largely concerned with the need and practical use of the appliance by the speakers. No research has been presented to prove that the arguments came from an analysis of the attitudes of wearers of the appliance. Furthermore, many of the psychological problems associated with loss of voice by laryngectomy are similar to those used against the use of an artificial larynx.

Some of the arguments are generalizations. For example, the statement that all persons can talk with an instrument does not stand up to the facts. Diedrich and Youngstrom point out that some people cannot or do not learn to use an instrument. Likewise the statement that the instrument is a distraction to the auditor and speaker does not agree with the experiences of auditors. We, ourselves, have never failed to understand a user of an artificial larynx in direct conversation or over the telephone, whereas we have often requested a poor esophageal speaker to repeat his statement. The statement that the instrument is not a good substitute for speech can be answered by calling attention to the many persons who have poor speech or no speech after laryngectomy.

The statement that first use of the artificial larynx will prevent the patient later from learning esophageal speech bears further discussion. Diedrich and Youngstrom stated that no one has ever proved this point. Furthermore, we know persons who first used an appliance extensively and later acquired esophageal speech. We once stubbornly and ignorantly refused to give esophageal speech therapy to a patient because he succumbed to a salesman's arguments and bought an appliance shortly after he left the hospital. When he was assigned for speech therapy, we indignantly informed him that if he were going to use the artificial larynx, there would be no need to teach esophageal speech. When we saw him some time later, he was talking exclusively with esophageal speech. The most interesting case we have on record is that of a man who was operated on in 1931, at which time he was given an artificial larynx. He became so adept with it that he was requested to join a scientific team that was demonstrating the latest discoveries in communication. His part was to demonstrate the pneumatic artificial larynx. In 1941 he heard a laryngectomee talk and decided he would talk that way. He became a proficient speaker without instruction. At this writing, he is 94 years of age, is still talking with esophageal speech and is active in Golden Age and church affairs. It might very well be assumed that his skill in articulation acquired by using the artificial larynx had made it easier for him to learn esophageal speech.

Usefulness of the Artificial Larynx

Serious consideration must be given to the use of an artificial larynx by patients who never learn to speak with esophageal voice. Should they be allowed to live the rest of their lives in silence, because of an unjustifiable attitude against the use of an appliance? Ample statistics have already been given to show that between two-fifths and one-third of laryngectomees do not learn to talk. A large proportion of these patients do not even gain the advantage of communication by an artificial larynx. For example, Putney reported that 32 per cent (140) of 440 patients never learned to talk, but only one-sixth of these used an appliance. This means that over 25 per cent of the total group communicated by whispers or writing. Horn found that only 29 per cent of nonspeakers use an appliance.

Additional arguments for early use of the artificial larynx may be found in favor of persons who require long times to learn esophageal speech. For example, Diedrich and Youngstrom; Horn, and Shames *et al.* reported that patients waited two or three months before they began speech instruction. Then it took four more months to acquire understandable esophageal speech. This means six or seven months to acquire proficiency. Diedrich and Youngstrom's patients took one year. Meanwhile these patients suffered with embarrassment and inconvenience because they could not communicate adequately. M.C.L. Greene and Heaver and Arnold state that lack of speech attainment or long delay in acquiring it may induce frustration and morbid preoccupation. This depression must be relieved by restoring the patient's ability to communicate.

Factors Affecting the Need for an Artificial Larynx

CHANGE IN PHYSICAL STRUCTURE. An aged person seldom has the drive and determination to conquer esophageal speech. He may be too feeble or unwilling to try, or his relatives may decide that he should use an appliance. Physical limitations may likewise prevent the patient's use of an instrument. Persons who have stenoses of the esophagus, esophagectomy, multiple handicaps, pharyngolaryngectomy, deafness, immobility of the tongue, loss of tissue or spasms of the cricopharyngeal muscle would not be classified as candidates for esophageal speech (Damsté; Diedrich and Youngstrom; M.C.L. Greene; Lanpher; Levin 1952, 1955; Pellegrini).

ENVIRONMENTAL CONDITIONS. The environment also can affect the patient's need for an appliance. If a factory worker has to converse under noisy conditions, or if greater volume is demanded than he can physically produce with esophageal voice (M.H. Miller), an appliance must be made available to him. Likewise, if a person becomes fatigued by using the telephone constantly, or if his weak voice does not carry well over the telephone, an appliance should solve his problem. Also, if a relative is hard of hearing, an appliance may give him better reception. The husband of one of our patients was hard of hearing and rejected his wife's attempt to speak because he couldn't understand her. She obtained an artificial larynx, an action which restored harmony to the family.

CONDITIONS OF EMPLOYMENT. The conditions under which laryngectomees work demand a study of their communication needs. Some patients make their own decisions before therapy is begun simply because they cannot otherwise work. An insurance salesman insisted on returning to work three weeks after surgery. He bought an artificial larynx before he took his first lesson. He successfully conducted his business until he retired. A supervisor of 300 draftsmen bought a device and returned to work one month after surgery. He never requested speech therapy. He believed he would lose his job if he returned without adequate communication; his superiors might decide that he was markedly limited in managing his staff. If she had not been advised to use an appliance shortly after surgery, a woman who had an esophagectomy would have had to wait in silence for more than six months while plastic surgery replaced the upper one-third of the esophagus and joined it to the pharynx.

Martin (1963) tells the tragic story of his patient who floundered for nine years because no one had shown him an artificial larynx. A president of a corporation was about to be asked for his resignation, the directors thinking he would not be able to direct the business. He bought an artificial larynx and was reelected. One man (Levin 1955) used an artificial larynx in his campaign for state senator and won. However, he was never happy with it, so he learned esophageal speech and later abandoned the aid. A salesman returned to work one month after surgery. Using an artificial larynx, he sold $35,000 worth of merchandise in one month. Meanwhile he worked on his speech and by the eighth month was able to communicate with his clients by esophageal speech.

Meeting Needs for Amplification

Laryngectomees who have weak voices, which must be heard during communication in business or in public addresses, obtain much benefit through amplification. The speaker holds at his lips a miniature microphone which is connected to a small chassis that is carried on his chest or held in his hand (Fig. 9). The chief complaints about most of the models that are available is the feedback which cannot be avoided because of the

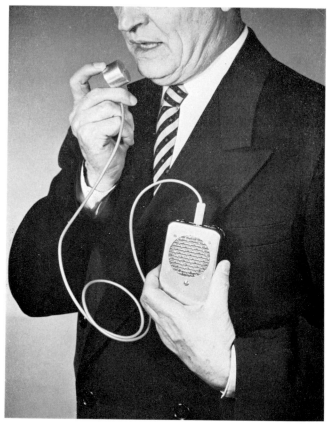

Figure 9. Rand Speech Amplifier with close-talking microphone. (*Courtesy of American Medical Association*)

proximity of the microphone to the speaker. However, users claim that they are satisfied if their weak voices are amplified enough to be heard. (See the Appendix for names of manufacturers.)

A bull horn, or electric megaphone (Fig. 10) has been used for talking to large audiences, especially out-of-doors. It is used by fire chiefs in directing their men at a fire. Policemen use it for crowd control. Using one, a laryngectomized marine officer was able to be heard the length of his lake ship. A minister used one for his revival meetings.

A portable rostrum molded in plastic frame, with a public address system built in, enables a laryngectomee to speak to a large group of people where a public address system is not available. It is also useful at Lost Chord Club meetings and conventions, and especially in schools. It is operated by battery and by alternating current. Local radio stores have them on display.

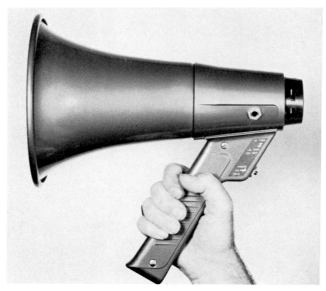

Figure 10. Power Page No. 2# electric megaphone for weak voices and crowd use (University Loudspeakers, Inc.). (*Courtesy of American Medical Association*)

Telephone Amplifiers. The Bell Telephone Company can modify the telephone so that the weak voice of a laryngectomee is amplified. A similar arrangement has also been used for some years to amplify the telephone receiver for a hard-of-hearing person.

When Should the Laryngectomee Be Shown the Artificial Larynx?

The artificial larynx may be routinely introduced to the patient prior to surgery or during the first or second interview (Diedrich and Youngstrom; McClear). It may also be loaned to the patient during the recovery period in the hospital (tube-in-the-mouth type), so that he can tell the staff how he feels (Irwin; Marge) and talk to relatives and friends (Heaver and Arnold; Luchsinger and Arnold). Likewise, the artificial larynx is demonstrated to the patient just before routine voice therapy is begun. The patient receives proof that he will always be able to talk, either by such an instrument or by esophageal speech (Diedrich and Youngstrom; M.C.L. Greene; Montreuil). These are all strategic moments. The last period may be the moment when the patient is expected or advised to decide whether he chooses to talk with esophageal voice or by means of an artificial larynx. According to some authorities, the decision should be the result of a mutual understanding and agreement by the laryngologist, speech clinician and patient (Diedrich and Youngstrom; Gardner 1961; M.C.L. Greene; Martin 1963). Another arrangement will be suggested later, in which the patient may be taught both methods of communication before he finally decides. After all that has been said, we should conclude by stating that some laryngectomees have not been able to talk with an artificial larynx (Diedrich and Youngstrom).

Chapter Five

PREPARING TO TEACH

WHEN SHOULD SPEECH THERAPY BE STARTED?

For purely psychological reasons, speech therapy should be begun as soon as possible after laryngectomy (M.C.L. Greene). Some therapists have suggested that speech therapy should begin two or three days after the nasogastric tube has been removed (Andrews; Fontaine and Mitchell; Jesberg; Kusske; Moolenaar-Bijl 1953b). This appears to be medically safe, since swallowing of liquids and foods without leakage indicates that the integrity of the PE segment has been established. Huber and Kopp recommended that it should begin "even if healing is not complete." Other authors, Chen *et al.*, stated that an occasional patient was started while the nasal tube was still being used, or before the postoperative fistula had closed.* We certainly do not see the urgency for, or the practicality of, such early therapy in light of our own and our contemporaries' experiences with fistulas that occurred after early speech therapy was given. For us, the fault lay in premature demonstration of esophageal speech; for the patients, the fault lay in unobserved, unanticipated and premature struggles to inject air. In order to prevent the development of fistulas, our surgeons recommend that speech therapy should begin two weeks after the patient leaves the hospital. An occasional healthy patient who has made an excellent recovery may be started on the day he is to leave the hospital. Other time criteria that have been suggested are two to four weeks after surgery (Diedrich and Youngstrom; Wintersteen) or six to eight weeks (Morrison). Keeping in mind that early initiation of speech is intended to insure successful therapy, we can point to Bondarenko's finding that 80 per cent of those who began therapy within two to five months after surgery acquired intelligible speech, whereas speech was attained by none of those who began therapy after 1½ to two years after surgery.

The discussion just concluded points to the use of two time factors: (a) when the wounds are soundly healed (Kallen; Morrison 1941) or during the latter part of the hospital stay (Waldrop and Baker), or (b) when

---

* No information was given about the techniques used to give speech therapy to the patient who still had a feeding tube in his nose. We would think that the patient would be so uncomfortable that he would refuse to cooperate!

the surgeon recommends that the patient is ready for speech therapy (Snidecor). The above schedules are also somewhat arbitrary because patients vary in recuperative powers and emotional stability. One of McCall's patients talked on the sixth postoperative day, immediately after the feeding tube was removed; another patient (female) talked on the tenth day. One of our patients, a 34-year-old male, said "Goodbye" as he left the hospital on the fourteenth day.

On the other hand, an occasional patient may have a stormy time during the postoperative period. As a result the surgeon gives him time to build up his health. Indeed, some patients are not made known to visitants or teachers for several months after surgery because they are in poor physical condition or are scheduled for a series of radiation treatments. Of course, speech therapy is withheld longest when a patient has an esophagectomy as well as a laryngectomy, followed by many months of skin grafting. As already pointed out, these patients should be given the use of an artificial larynx permanently or until they are ready for speech therapy. M.C.L. Greene considers that it is advantageous for future speech success to permit the patient who has a fistula or who has a feeding tube retained longer than usual to visit a speech class. He is not then allowed to attempt speech, but hopefully his tension and anxiety are replaced by a relaxed assurance that he, too, will be successful when he starts speech class.

WHO SHOULD TEACH ESOPHAGEAL SPEECH?

A Conflict of Opinion

Considerable emotion has been displayed by both laryngectomized speech teachers and speech pathologists in regard to their respective capabilities (or privileges) to train the laryngectomee to speak. Most laryngectomees argue that they have a special affinity (Baker), a bond (Berry and Eisenson) or a unique contribution to make (Nessel) with laryngectomees because having had a laryngectomy, they understand the problems that have to be faced and conquered.* Mary Doehler, a laryngectomee and teacher of many hundreds of patients, insists that the teacher should be a laryngectomized person. Laryngectomees also say that the patient is at a disadvantage with a speech pathologist who can only demonstrate a word or two. (Hollyfield). Lanpher, a laryngectomized teacher who taught French in a high school before and after her laryngectomy, says that we cannot be dogmatic. She knows some effective laryngectomized teachers who are dynamic and flexible. Specific training is necessary for either type

---

* See Lauder's presentation of the opposing arguments (Lauder 1965).

of teacher, but even this is not enough. She states that a successful teacher is one who can project what she knows, and who has the ability to inspire or motivate others to want to learn, explore and improve. Either type of teacher must have these important qualities. (Lanpher 1965).

Several laryngologists state that the laryngectomized person needs the help of those who have had to learn esophageal speech themselves (Clark; Equen 1965; Pitkin). Johnson observed that the first two hundred patients in his hospital who were treated by a lay teacher had as good speech as those who were trained by a speech pathologist. However, he did not indicate how the speech of these patients was evaluated. Corgill agreed with this statement, adding that he could not see how a speech therapist can convince a depressed patient that he will be able to speak, when he himself (the therapist or laryngologist) is unable to demonstrate adequate esophageal speech. Martin (1963) also prefers a lay teacher who can inspire the patient into believing that by persistent effort he can learn to speak again. Moses, a phonetician and laryngologist, opposes the view of his colleagues because he believes that the teacher is not equipped to handle complicated problems. Damsté thinks it best to leave teaching to experts who are trained rather than to those who have undergone a laryngectomy.

Almost no speech pathologists recommend that a laryngectomized instructor be the sole adviser and teacher of a laryngectomee except under special conditions, for example, where there is no one else in the area to do the work. Ferguson agrees with this exception because large areas may have no professionally trained people. It was logical for Curran, who found no teacher available in her area and who was forced to learn esophageal speech without instruction, to become an enthusiastic and successful teacher and to organize a Lost Chord Club. This has repeatedly occurred with trainees from the IAL institutes.

Speech pathologists complain that the larygectomized teacher knows and teaches only the method he uses (Snidecor). We recall that several laryngectomized trainees at one of the early IAL institutes terminated their training in different methods of teaching with the remark, "All I know is that I can swallow air, and that's what I am going to teach." Waldrop proved by cinematographic x-ray that one laryngectomee who claimed he swallowed air for speech and taught that technique actually used the tongue press or injection method (Waldrop and Baker). Success in learning a skill is not a criterion of the ability to teach (Keenan). Others assert that a lay teacher without specific training in organic pathology can jeopardize a patient's future (Knox; Ross). Hyman (1965) observed that the lay instructor does not use step-by-step procedures and may not follow ethical procedures relative to the patient, family and physicians. One such teacher thought that he had become an expert on intimate relationships between a laryngectomee and his spouse! Moore (1965) stated that a laryngectomee who loses his larynx is not the most desirable person to teach others who lose the larynx any more than a man who loses a leg is the best person to teach an amputee to walk.

The present discussion reminds us of a similar situation that arose thirty years ago in the history of lip reading instruction. The only early teachers of lip reading had been hard-of-hearing persons. They wrote textbooks on the subject. Many of the directors of the Leagues for the Hard of Hearing were hard of hearing themselves. One director, who was advising a client on the selection of a hearing aid was heard to say: "Well, I use _____ hearing aid." Today, directors of speech and hearing centers, successors to the leagues, are speech pathologists. Professionally trained therapists with normal hearing teach lip reading methods in the public schools and colleges. Likewise, deaf teachers of deaf students are being replaced by college-trained teachers who hear normally.

How Can We Resolve This Conflict?

Berlin (1965b), a speech pathologist, resolves the conflict by saying that he would not be biased, provided the teacher had deep sensitivity for the feelings of the patient, a sound knowledge in the field in which he is working, personal integrity and intelligence. However, he qualifies this opinion by saying that scientifically, "laryngectomees are in better hands if they stay with proficiently trained people who have the capacity to advance technical knowledge scientifically and systematically." A general agreement among speech pathologists and some laryngectomees (Behringer; Corgill; Mawhinney; Ross; Stoll) gives the laryngectomized person a definite, important place on the rehabilitation team. They agree that an intelligent, "psychologically astute" (Stoll 1965) laryngectomee who learns good speech can be a great support in the preoperative and postoperative stages in building morale and in showing the patient that he can lead an essentially normal life (Knox). Likewise, he may be of great value in demonstrating esophageal speech at different levels of recovery (Snidecor 1965). Levin (1965) says that an excellent combination is the lay teacher demonstrating for a speech pathologist. Shanks claims that there is enough room to combine forces toward a common goal of helping laryngectomees, "rather than fighting each other."

The value of training both kinds of teachers has been demonstrated by the IAL, who obtained financial support for voice institutes from the Office of Vocational Rehabilitation and the American Cancer Society. Members of the American Speech and Hearing Association and laryngectomized teachers from the IAL gave the institutes a capable staff of consultants and instructors (Fig. 11). Half of the trainees were speech pathologists. Preference was given to laryngectomees who lived in areas where there was no voice instruction. The IAL has published a list of laryngectomized teachers who have answered the requirements of experience and adequate training, and the American Speech and Hearing Association has published a list of its members who are in a position to teach esophageal speech.

The criteria for teachers of esophageal speech that have been offered by different writers (Laguaite; Lanpher 1965; Lauder; Martin 1963; Shanks; Snidecor 1965; Stoll 1965; Van Riper and Irwin) resemble the criteria that are required of teachers of almost any subject in almost any institution. In other words, the therapist should be patient, flexible, imaginative, intelligent, sympathetic and understanding, with personal integrity, a deep sensitivity for the feelings of the patient and the ability to motivate and inspire. In addition, the teacher should have a background in anatomy, phonetics, psychology, physiology and other subjects that will permit him

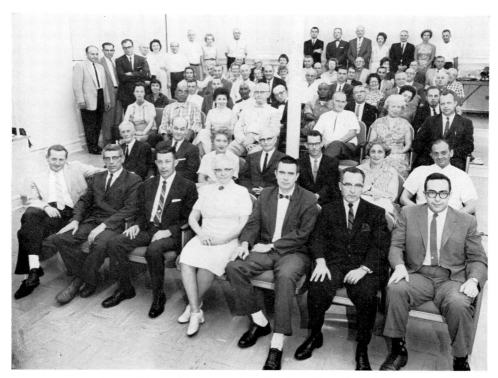

Figure 11. Members of Second Institute for Teaching Esophageal Speech, held under auspices of IAL and Office of Vocational Rehabilitation, School of Medicine, Memphis, Tennessee, Medical Center. About half of the group are laryngectomees. (*Courtesy of Les Cooper*)

to convey clearly the principles of producing esophageal speech and help the patient adapt to his changed situation. Shames *et al.* also recommended a way that is acceptable to both groups by stating: "The laryngectomee needs a competent teacher who is proficient in esophageal processes, general learning processes, and who can provide proper motivation."

We do not know to what extent the above criteria are possessed by professional and lay teachers of esophageal speech. If the latter have not attended an institute, they may not possess all the criteria. We do know, however, that both types of teachers are sharing about equally in the work with laryngectomees. The 1969 *Directory* of IAL lists ninety-nine speech pathologists and 109 lay teachers who are teaching laryngectomees in the clubs of the Association. It appears that the laryngectomized patient has won this argument, because both types of teachers are contributing substantially to his speech rehabilitation.

ANTICIPATED ACHIEVEMENT IN ESOPHAGEAL SPEECH

Before we begin speech therapy for laryngectomized persons, it would be profitable to determine, or to anticipate, what goals should be used and to what extent a group of laryngectomized persons can reach them. This information should enable us to build our teaching program in keeping with acceptable levels of achievement and in stages that the experiences of others have shown to be successful.

We have very little information on percentages of achievement at different levels that a given population of patients may achieve. We thought that we might obtain such a percentage distribution from a group of forty laryngectomees who were at a club meeting. The number of their postoperative years varied from two to twenty. They were requested to raise their hands if the described level of speech efficiency fitted their own abilities. Using the Barton-Hejna Scale, and starting at the lowest level, No Sounds Produced, we described each succeeding level. No hands were raised until the next to the best level, Good Use of Sentences, was described, when two hands appeared. The rest of the group raised their hands promptly in answer to the level, Fluent Nonhesitant Speech. In that group were speakers who used two and three seconds or gulped two or three times before they injected air. Others were often asked to repeat their conversation when they were not understood. The rate of speaking of some members was low and the voices of others were weak. One member used an instrument when the speaking situation was difficult. This surprising response indicated that most esophageal speakers appear to be satisfied with a low level of speech attainment. They apparently are not sensitive to their own speech inaccuracies or to reports from their own self-monitoring equipment. Their therapists may not have developed this sensitivity, and, because of advancing age, some patients may not have heard their own speech to evaluate it. Wepman *et al.* states: "Many patients discontinue their efforts to obtain satisfactory esophageal speech because they cannot visualize their progress." Heaver *et al.* put the percentage of discouraged patients at 40 per cent. It is thus common knowledge that far too many patients either are dismissed or have withdrawn from instruction before reaching a high level of proficiency.

Percentages of Achievement in a Population of Laryngectomees

A few percentage distributions of patients at different levels of speech achievement have been gleaned from the literature, or have been calculated by us from the meager information that was obtainable. Freud divided his group of fifty-five patients according to the following grades of speech skill: excellent, 18.2 per cent; good, 52.7 per cent; fair, 20 per cent; inadequate or no speech, 9.1 per cent. Diedrich and Youngstrom's sixty-eight speakers, answering questionnaires, rated their own speech as follows: good or very good, 56 per cent; average, 23 per cent; fair, 11 per cent; poor, 10 per cent. Fourteen users of the artificial larynx rated themselves as follows: very good or good, 67 per cent; average, 17 per cent; fair, 5 per cent; poor, 11 per cent. Fifty per cent of Jackson's patients evaluated their speech as being good.

Speech clinicians have classified speech achievement levels in terms of language facility or various aspects of speech and voice. Robe *et al.* (1956a) used the following classification:

	No.	*Per Cent**
1. No sounds produced	1	3.1
2. Partial control; single sounds under fair control	1	3.1
3. Simple words produced	2	6.2
4. Combined two and three words	2	6.2
5. Some sentences used	1	3.1
6. Sentences consistently used	7	22.0
7. Fluent nonhesitant speech	18	56.3
	32	100.0

* Our calculation of percentages.

From levels 6 and 7, we found that 78.3 per cent of the patients used consistent sentences or fluent speech, and 3 per cent used some sentences. Gardner (1964) obtained a slightly smaller percentage, 77.5 per cent of patients with adequate speech from 115 working laryngectomees who rated their own speech abilities.

Using three levels of achievement, Damsté found that 26 per cent had serviceable speech and 70 per cent had good or excellent speech. On the basis of the criteria Loud Enough To Be Intelligible and Devoid of All Discordant Elements, Martin (1963) stated that only a small percentage of laryngectomees would qualify for adequate speech.

Judges of Berlin's (1965a) study of the speech abilities of sixty-two laryngectomees who attended an IAL convention used the following criteria for evaluating speech adequacy: intelligibility, clarity of articulation, relaxed sound without strain, fluency in going from phrase to phrase and lack of air or stoma noise. Their findings produced the following percentages: very good speech, 48.4 per cent; acceptable speech, 22.6 per cent; poor speech, 19.3 per cent; not acceptable, 9.7 per cent.* It is seen that only 72 per cent of this group had adequate speech.

Besides the descriptive terms used by Berlin, other writers (Darley; Moore 1953; Snidecor 1968; Sparks) offered rate of talking; ease of speaking; good continuity; polished phrasing; adequate pitch inflection; adequate loudness; no consciousness of swallowing or eructation; coordination of voice production with vegetative breathing; harsh, husky, wet, dry qualities, and evidence of great effort. However, no percentage distributions were available for rating the efficiency of the voices.

A most useful rating method was offered by Wepman *et al.* as a result of experience in evaluating the efficiency of his patients. He used a combination of sound production and speech efficiency:

Level	Esophageal Sounds Produced	Speech Efficiency
7	None	No speech
6	Involuntary sound only	No speech
5	Voluntary sound part of time	No speech
4	Voluntary sound part of time	Vowel sounds differentiated; monosyllabic speech
3	Voluntary sounds at will	Single word speech
2	Voluntary sounds at will, with continuity	Word grouping
1	Automatic speech	Esophageal speech

This scale, like that of Robe *et al.*, can be used to classify the speech achievement of a group of patients or to indicate the level that a patient has reached at a given time. Wepman's scale also has the advantage of separating sound production from speech production. This gives the teacher a much more detailed picture of a patient's achievement.

Berlin (1963a) developed a scale that is based on the probable rate of growth of basic skills in terms of time required. It was developed in the process of determining the rate of growth of veterans, who were kept

* Our calculation of percentages.

under rigidly controlled instruction, three times a day, while they stayed in a Veterans Administration hospital:

1. Ability to phonate on demand twenty times:
    Among good speakers, 100 per cent attained the skill in ten to fourteen days.
    Among poor speakers, 68 per cent attained the skill in twenty-four days.
2. Short latency period between injection and phonation:
    Good speakers reached an average of 0.24 second by twentieth day.
    Poor speakers reached an average of 1.3 seconds by twentieth day.
3. Sustaining a vowel for adequate duration:
    Good speakers reached an average of 2.8 seconds by eighteenth day.
    Poor speakers reached an average of 1.3 seconds by eighteenth day.
4. Number of plosive syllables produced on one inflation:
    Good speakers reached an average of 8.6 by twenty-fifth day.
    Poor speakers reached an average of 2.3 by twenty-fifth day.

Although the time factors are not totally accurate because some of the patients missed lessons, we consider the scale to be valuable for two reasons: (a) it comprises skills that are most essential for effective esophageal speech, and (b) it gives us criteria for comparing the growth of patients in terms of time. However, we must point out that the time factor was exaggerated for average comparisons because of accelerated teaching. In the quiet, relaxed speech clinic, patients would be expected to learn the skills in quantities of weeks rather than days. We favor instruction in frequent, concentrated periods, daily or several times a week. Furthermore, when group instruction is a routine procedure, special, individual lessons should be given to those who have difficulties in acquiring some basic skills. Under such circumstances, the rate of achievement would vary with the frequency and nature of the therapy.

Graduated Stages of Speech Development

Although the achievement and rating scales mentioned above have given us useful information on the classification of populations of laryngectomees, we need more specific details about growth and how it can be developed. Diedrich and Youngstrom; M.C.L. Greene, and Snidecor have listed stages in teaching esophageal speech. All of these methods should be studied in great detail because they are effective in developing the esophageal sound, and these authors agree that the peculiar nature of the plosive consonant should be used to initiate the esophageal sound. Diedrich and Youngstrom offer several optional techniques for doing this, thereby maintaining their policy of using an eclectic approach. M.C.L. Greene and Snidecor have listed detailed steps of the development of esophageal speech which agree quite closely except for additional procedures offered by Greene. Snidecor's (1968) nine stages are logically arranged for developing esophageal speech from the first speech sound to fluently delivered speech:

1. Get air in, get air out.
2. Produce consonants (plosives), vowels and diphthongs.
3. Voice simple, useful, one-syllable words.
4. Voice two-syllable words—at first with one air-charge per syllable then with one air-charge for both syllables.
5. Voice simple phrases with one charge if possible.
6. Practice articulation and connected speech with emphasis on (a) vowels, (b) diphthongs and (c) consonants.
7. Stress is achieved by changes in loudness, pitch, quality and time.
8. Use active conversation.
9. The achievement of a satisfactory rate usually results along with the mastery of the previous eight stages.

The additional stage that M.C.L. Greene offers is relaxation and breathing as a preliminary procedure to formal presentation of plosive sounds. She also includes exercises such as whistling and blowing a mouth organ, and other devices to develop diaphragmatic and thoracic movements (Hodson and Oswald's techniques). We also believe in relaxation and breathing techniques which are intended to prepare the patient for an easy, relaxed state of mind and body, just as we have found them helpful with all other types of voice patients.

Proposed Plans for Developing Esophageal Speech

Periodic Achievement Tests

We propose to set up a series of tests that will measure the acquisition of certain skills from time to time as a means of demonstrating progress. These will be similar to the skills tested in Berlin's series: phonation, latency and duration of vowels and syllable. Another test will include the rate of reading aloud a given passage. Spaces will be arranged for periodic tests which will serve as an indication of progress and as a stimulus to the patient to keep working to improve his speech. We hope that these tests will be used by speech clinicians, and that they will discover their value in raising the percentage of patients in a given population that attains a level of good or excellent speech. Instructions to clinicians to give the periodic tests are spaced throughout the series. The entire battery is located in Chapter 6.

Phases of Instruction

The formal instruction for developing esophageal speech is based on twenty-five years of clinical experience, and on observation of the techniques of contemporaries practiced at numerous teaching sessions during IAL institutes and conventions. The instruction is divided into seven phases, which begin with a preliminary probing of the ability of the patient to produce an esophageal sound by any or all methods. This is followed by formal attempts to develop the esophageal sound by the prevailing methods, aided by clinical techniques adapted to each method.

Efforts are next directed toward improving sustained pressure of air in order to prolong vowels and to increase the number of sounds and syllables per air-charge. The final phases will be devoted to developing fluency, restoring the melody in the voice and increasing intelligibility. Following the formal instruction by phases, a special section will be devoted to group speech therapy. The final section on instruction in esophageal speech contains numerous suggestions and techniques that are useful for supplementing the material in the formal instruction, and for solving the problems of difficult cases.

EVALUATION OF THE LARYNGECTOMEE

A practical approach to teaching postlaryngectomy speech requires an extensive evaluation of the patient soon after his operation. It is necessary to determine his assets and liabilities, and to know what limitations might affect his progress in the development of speech. It is also important to determine how much he has changed from his previous physical condition. Evaluation may begin as early as the preoperative interview with the patient, and may continue throughout the immediate and convalescent postoperative periods, during which time the speech clinician on the hospital-clinic staff may see the patient many times. Other speech clinicians, on the other hand, may see the patient for the first time only after the surgeon has referred him for speech instruction. In the former situation, the clinician is fortunate because from the very beginning of the patient's hospitalization he will begin to assemble information that is pertinent to a fairly intelligent prognosis for speech achievement. The clinician who sees the patient when he is ready for speech instruction may have to utilize several sources to obtain the necessary medical information and background about the patient before he can plan an intelligent program of therapy (Knepflar). In either situation, the speech clinician considers it fortunate if he has the patient's background and history available for planning rehabilitation.

Knepflar has compiled a most complete list of the factors that should be evaluated before therapy starts, and Johnson has prepared a complete case history for a laryngectomy. As they point out, it is necesary to ascertain what factors indicate the probability of a routine therapeutic program and what factors indicate individual difficulties that will require special handling. One of the first and most important factors is the medical and surgical history of the patient.

Surgical Factors

The date of surgery is deemed critical if the patient begins speech therapy many months later. The longer the interval of time after surgery, the less are the chances for attaining adequate speech (Damsté; Harrington, Laguaite). Damsté believes that under favorable conditions, good esophageal speech is almost completely realized in the first year. Others have observed that patients continue to improve their speech for an average of two years after surgery (Diedrich and Youngstrom; Horn). We know one surgeon, a laryngectomee, who kept records of his voice for five years. His speech increased in fluency and intelligibility from year to year. Perhaps we should argue that provided the patient has the determination to achieve it, anyone who decides to begin speech therapy within two years will have a greater chance of attaining good speech than one who begins therapy after two years.

We have found very few people who began therapy more than two years after surgery. At that late date, they were not willing or interested or inspired to attempt to begin speech therapy. They usually had settled into a groove where speech demands were minimal and social contacts were few. We had one exception to this type of situation, a patient who quit after three lessons but returned a year later with the determination to learn to talk. As a hair stylist in a sophisticated community, he quickly found how important it was to talk about the newest hair styles in an enthusiastic manner. He finished his course only after off-and-on attendance for six months.

The speech clinician takes special notice of any type of surgery that may prevent, discourage or delay the early acquisition of speech. Thus, the patient who endures months of plastic surgery or extensive radiation therapy, or whose loss of, or damage to, tissue or presence of scars prevents dilatation or relaxation of the esophageal sphincter (PE segment or PE junction) (Bangs *et al.;* Damsté), may experience long periods of silence. Likewise, a fistula or stenosis (Chen *et al.*) may require use of a feeding tube which prolongs silence during the healing period. It also may increase anxiety and embarrassment to such a degree that the patient becomes completely discouraged about seeking speech therapy. (We have already suggested that such a person may use an artificial larynx, with permission of the surgeon.) The clinician also would like to know what muscles have been excised or have lost function because of severance of the nerve supply, as in radical resections (M.C.L. Greene).

However, there is a difference of opinion regarding the effects of the severity of surgery upon acquisition of speech. For example, Snidecor quoted Stern as believing that the new voice is dependent upon the anatomical conditions created during the operation. Yet Putney later stated that removal of all or part of the hyoid cartilage did not make any difference in speech efficiency and that the types of incisions had no effect on voice. The loss of tissue in the pharynx, hypopharynx and cervical esophagus did not have much effect on voice acquisition. Likewise, he stated that the 38 per cent of his patients who did not learn to talk had no outstanding anatomical reason for their failures. Furthermore, Seeman in 1958 stated:

> The various methods of operation themselves have no influence upon the functional results of esophageal speech. After all, the site of the operation lies above the mouth of the esophagus. It is only necessary to preserve the cricopharyngeal muscle and not to destroy its innervation provided by the recurrent nerve.

Diedrich and Youngstrom's spot x-ray and cinefluorographic studies of areas and dimensions of the reconstructed hypopharynx and the PE segment revealed no significant relationship between surgery or x-ray treatment and successful speech.* Snidecor, summing up the results of his study, stated that the type of surgery—for example, removal of the strap muscles—did not appear to determine the relative excellence of the voice or the extent of required speech training. Studies of Shames *et al.* agreed with Snidecor's findings.

These differences of opinion serve as a warning to the voice clinician that he should not always attribute failure of voice therapy to the anatomical changes that result from surgery. Rather, he should evaluate his own understanding and treatment of the patient. However, it is obvious that he must have at hand all available information on physical changes

---

* Read Diedrich and Youngstrom's list of physical and psychological factors that may prevent learning of speech.

in the muscles and organs that are concerned with the production of esophageal voice, in order to utilize the patient's residual complex of muscle and organ function to develop as proficient esophageal speech as is possible.

Physical Factors

Good general physical condition and health are supportive factors in enabling the patient to initiate and maintain adequate speech. Knepflar; Laguaite, and Snidecor emphasize the need to treat the whole man. Although this is not solely the speech clinician's responsibility, he should be aware of negative factors, known or controlled by surgeons and other professional persons, that may defeat his therapeutic program; hence, he must assay the possibilities of compensating for them.

Some patients who have strong, sturdy bodies and healthy mental attitudes go through their surgical and postoperative experiences in a routine, problem-free manner. Surgeons do not hesitate to send these patients to a voice teacher immediately after discharge from the hospital. Other patients have stormy times not only because of extensive surgery but because they are in a debilitated state and remain so for some time after recovery from surgery (Bangs *et al.;* M.C.L. Greene; Morrison). Likewise, it is not at all rare for a laryngectomized person to be a chronic alcoholic or a postalcoholic who has become addicted to drugs. These patients may not be amenable to voice therapy because of self-concern, lack of willpower and inability to persist until sucessful speech is attained. We know of several laryngectomees who accepted the bottle as their sole companion and source of comfort. On the other hand, we have seen patients who had earlier joined Alcoholics Anonymous display the same determination to succeed in speech that they had shown in overcoming chronic, debilitating alcoholism. They have eagerly and faithfully visited alcoholic laryngectomees in the hospitals and at home with the hope that they might persuade them to regain their self-respect and self-control.

It is always important to obtain information about past histories of gastric and duodenal ulcers. The sheer shock of surgery and the exposure of the alimentary tract to spontaneous intake of air may reactivate the old ulcer. In addition, the repetitive effort to take in air by the swallow or even a forceful modified swallow may move so much air into the stomach that the patient will have to cease all therapy until the ulcer heals again (Gardner, 1956, 1961). These personal observations have been verified in conversation with contemporary speech pathologists and surgeons.

Geriatric Factors

Since the highest incidence of cancer of the larynx is among persons who are in their seventh decade of life, the clinician should anticipate that the generally weak patient may not have the energy to persist and may tire quickly in his efforts to develop speech adequacy (Harrington). Some of our patients who were in their seventies simply wrote that they were too old to learn, or their relatives decided that "an electro-larynx would be easier for Dad." Several of our oldest patients who were encouraged by visitations to start speech therapy quit after two or three lessons with the remark, "It isn't worth the effort." Other patients of similar ages who had developed and maintained their physical stamina and mental alertness after years of competition in business had little trouble in learning speech. Damsté believes that there is "some connection between speech and age which has an adverse influence on persons in the ages of sixty and sixty-five and older." Our own studies and those of others (Table II) show a consistent decline in the percentage of

TABLE II
PERCENTAGES OF SPEECH SUCCESS BY AGE GROUPS

Perello (1956)		Smith et al.		Svane-Knudson		Gardner (1966)	
Age Range	Per Cent Success	Age Range	Per Cent Success	Age Range	Per Cent Success	Age Range	Per Cent Success
20–40	88	21–40	—	21–40	—	21–40	100
41–60	56	41–50	87	41–50	89.3	40–60	75
61–75	30	51–60	80	51–60	72.2	—	—
—	—	61–	49	61–	50.0	61–	50

speech success with age. The younger the patients, the higher the number who acquire adequate speech. The older they are, the fewer are the chances for attaining adequate speech. Diedrich and Youngstrom, however, found no relationship between chronological age and speech skill with a small number of cases. However, Harrington states that the older patients are slower to recuperate and slower in requesting instruction, and that slower recovery means longer periods of silence which influence habits of communication that must be changed by the therapist.

With age also come frailty (M.C.L. Greene; Harrington; Morrison 1941), general debility (Brodnitz) and lack of energy or persistence (Bangs *et al.;* Long). Diedrich and Youngstrom; and Vrticka and Svoboda found no relationship between arthritic changes and speech skill, but Weihs' poorer speakers had greater arthritic changes than the better speakers. Flaccidity of muscles (Lanpher) makes it harder to learn speech. Other conditions, such as degeneration (Long), senility (Diedrich and Youngstrom), arteriosclerosis with memory lapse (Diedrich and Youngstrom), cardiovascular and cerebrovascular conditions (Long) and apraxia or inability to imitate motor skills (Diedrich and

Youngstrom), make it difficult even to begin therapy. Damsté states that persons who are past 60 years of age are slower in their rate of speech, are unable to monitor voice quality and are indifferent to the pitch of the voice. These weaknesses doubtless are related to a decrease in auditory reception (Bangs *et al.;* Diedrich and Youngstrom; Lanpher 1965) which prevents the patient from monitoring his speech. According to Diedrich and Youngstrom, the greater the hearing loss, the poorer the speech. (Hence, every patient should have a sensory and speech threshold test.) In addition, deafness of close relatives with subsequent misunderstandings discourages the patient's effort to make himself understood. Contributing to the last factor may be dental health (Long; Snidecor) and eventual mastication problems.

The speech clinician is thus forewarned about factors that affect the learning ability of older persons. It is a challenge to him to hold the patient's interest and to inspire him to persist to successful speech. Heaver *et al.* offer a word of caution here that older persons may continue to come to the teacher or to the clubs, which are islands of security for them. Thus, a dependency relationship may be perpetuated rather than complete rehabilitation. We noticed this tendency among the aged hard of hearing who sought association with hard-of-hearing persons and relaxation and perhaps shelter in the former leagues for the hard of hearing.

Psychological Factors

Emotional Problems

In the section on preoperative orientation, we emphasized the traumatic reality of cancer and the impending loss of the larynx. In preparing to give speech therapy, the speech clinician must know the ultimate result of these reactions, that is, the direction which the patient has taken in preparing himself not only for speech therapy but for the many adjustments that loss of normal speech demands. He must know the strength of the patient's desire to learn speech and whether he is to have his full cooperation (Damsté). In other words, the speech clinician must consider how he can capitalize on the factors that favor restoration of speech, and how he can alter the unfavorable forces that might defeat his goals.

The speech clinician who has repeatedly seen the patient during convalescence may already have evaluated the personality factors. He may have observed that one group of patients consists of introverted, brooding, withdrawn, depressed or anxious persons (Damsté; Gardner 1966; Luchsinger and Arnold). The patients' esthetic sensitivity to altered breathing and feeding and to scarring may have produced feelings of inferiority and rejection as well as loss of self-esteem (Damsté; Gardner 1966; M.C.L. Greene; Howie; Knepflar; Luchsinger and Arnold). They may already have given up hope of learning a new type of speaking. In another group of patients, the clinician may find extroverted, aggressive, outgoing, self-confident persons (Long; Snidecor) who have already mastered numerous life-situations and whose self-discipline, tenacity and courage can carry them through the vicissitudes of laryngectomies (Bisi and Conley; M.C.L. Greene; Putney).

Horn found that self-discipline and determination were the most important factors in learning esophageal speech. Damsté admitted that he had seen only one truly depressed patient among his laryngectomees. It is obvious, therefore, that the speech clinician must be able to distinguish unfavorable reactions from the normal, expected reactions to a handicap, such as the fears and anxieties of the unknown to which well-adjusted persons will eventually adapt themselves. To paraphrase the writing of the well-known war reporter Ernie Pyle, the well adjusted person may be scared but not afraid.

Motivation

A clinician need not go far into his evaluation before he decides if the patient is highly motivated and should regain adequate speech and return to his former milieu. One such motive is economic pressure to earn a living for his family (Darley; Horn; Kusske; Long; Snidecor). Horn found that "necessity for earning a living" was the second most important factor in learning esophageal speech. Another motive is a strong desire to succeed in speech in order to regain prestige among friends and business associates (Damsté *et al.*) The clinician may rejoice when an elderly man states that he wants to be able to talk to his grandchildren. A grandmother confidently explains that she wants to have a new voice as a Christmas present for her loved ones, and so that she can babysit again.

The speech clinician can also sense early in his evaluation if the patient has already made up his mind that he will not talk and does not wish to return to his friends. This revelation points out a prospective difficult patient because laryngectomees who react unfavorably, for example, to their surgical scars and stomas, or who decide to avoid their friends, are less likely to regain intelligible speech, if they do at all, than those who react favorably to the same condition or who gladly seek their friends (Gardner 1966).*

* For additional information on psychological problems of laryngectomees, consult Bisi and Conley; Damsté; Diedrich and Youngstrom; Fontaine and Mitchell; Gardner 1966; Klieger; Levin; Long; Luchsinger and Arnold; Martin 1963; Moses; Nahum and Golden; Pitkin; Schall 1954; Shanks; and Stoll.

Intelligence

Very few claims have been made that lack of intelligence contributes to failure to learn esophageal speech. Chen *et al.* and Morrison believe that poor learning ability may impede the acquisition of esophageal speech. For example, the patient may lack the insight to understand and master coordination of a new muscular action (DiCarlo *et al.;* M.C.L. Greene). We do find an occasional patient who appears to be unable to follow simple directions or who continues to use a habit that other patients usually alter quite promptly. One of our patients kept blowing violently from his stoma. Upon trying to converse with him, an older club member remarked, "H_____, man, why don't you stop that blowing?" It took him over a year to break the habit.

Damsté states that no particular amount of intelligence is required for a patient to learn a new type of speaking, but he feels that a quick mind and the ability to recognize kinesthetic sensations help a person to overcome anatomical or functional difficulties. However, Seeman (1967) quotes Nemec and Vrticka as having found a significant correlation between quality of voice and intelligence. M.C.L. Greene barely touches on intelligence when she says,

> Application of the basic principles related to air intake into the vicarious lung must develop along lines favorable to the patient's learning ability and his anatomical and physiological possibilities.

These arguments point up the problems of the examining speech clinician. He will be able to confirm his earlier impressions of the patient's learning capacity as he continues to teach him. If there is a real problem in learning, a brief intelligence test will enable the clinician to alter his teaching program according to his findings.

Social Factors

If the patient lives alone, the speech clinician can predict that the patient will not achieve adequate speech unless special arrangements are made. Such a person does not receive the stimulation and encouragement of a family. Hence, he has less need to talk and less need to learn (Harrington; Horn; Lanpher 1965; Long). He needs someone to urge him to get away from the television set and to work on speech. Lanpher (1965) states that it is much harder for a lone person to learn to talk. "When you are learning to talk there is a period in which you need someone to talk to." (See also Harrington; and Long.) It is even worse when a patient is rejected by members of the family. For example, 46 per cent of husbands and 60 per cent of single women's relatives did not give moral support to laryngectomized women (Gardner 1966). It is very fortunate, on the other hand, to learn that the majority of the spouse's relatives were sympathetic and supported the patients' efforts to talk (Darley; Gardner 1966; Horn; Snidecor).

We know numerous wives and husbands who have patiently urged, or arranged for, the patients to work persistently on their speech. Sons, daughters, grandchildren, brothers and sisters rooted for one of our patients, and rejoiced when he learned to talk. However, an unhealthy family influence, such as one where there is excessive sympathy and solicitude, may place the patient in a position of dependency from which he may not acquire suitable esophageal speech (Diedrich and Youngstrom; Knepflar; Laguaite; Horn found that encouragement of the family was the third most important factor in learning speech. It is therefore important for the clinician to interview as many relatives that come to his attention as he can in order to discern the extent of their interest (or lack of it) in the welfare of the patient. He then must incorporate in his plans ways and means of supplementing this important shortcoming (Harrington; Horn; Lanpher 1965; Long). He must persuade relatives or friends to encourage the patient to work on his speech. It is obvious that one of the speech clinician's tasks is to educate not only individuals but also the general public on the problems and needs of the laryngectomized person.

Malfunctions of the New Speech Mechanism

Flexibility of the Neoglottis

To determine how well a person can swallow, it is first necessary to ask him if he has had any difficulty in eating, specifically in swallowing food. If he reports that he can swallow the average sizes of solid foods, such as small chunks of meat, peanuts, crackers and dry cereal (Snidecor) or hard candies without lodging them in the hypopharynx or in the upper esophagus, he should have adequate function of the PE segment, as well as normal peristaltic action. He also should be able to take air in for communication by esophageal speech. Stetson (1937b) stated that if a patient can swallow satisfactorily, he can learn to talk. On the other hand, if the patient has to chew food into a fine, smooth condition, or if he has to eat puréed or finely cut foods (the spouse can help with this information), or if food particles lodge in his throat or are moved only by swallowing liquids, we may suspect that the narrowness of the PE segment may prevent quick learning of adequate air-charge. Damsté reported that patients who had swallowing difficulties and had a tight sphincter were limited to a pharyngeal type of speech. The wisest thing to do is to discuss the problem with the laryngologist.

The speech clinician may test the efficiency of the neoglottis by asking the patient to swallow chunky items like whole peanut halves, candy jelly beans, coarse, dry cereal or raisins* (Snidecor). By placing his fingers on the neck over the path of the esophagus, the speech clinician can detect the peristaltic action as the food particles, air or liquid move downward. Of course, the most practical test is to instruct the patient to swallow air and to observe the promptness of the patient's attempts. If the bolus is moved downward only after marked delay, or if the air is finally explosively squeezed downward, it may indicate that the neoglottic muscles are controlled by an excessively strong contraction (Damsté). It is likely that the patient will have difficulty in overcoming neoglottic action for injecting air for esophageal speech. In such cases, the speech clinician will make a note that the laryngologist should be consulted regarding the possible need of dilating or relaxing the overly tense musculature of the esophagus.

Contrasted with adequate function and overcontraction of the lumen of the esophagus is an abnormally flabby or open mouth. This, of course, cannot be evaluated by the swallowing test; rather the absence of the closure may be roughly determined by requesting the patient to take in a mouthful of water, tilt his head back and let the water pour into the pharynx without swallowing it. Several patients were unable to hold the water because it appeared to descend at once into the esophagus. One patient discovered that he could inhale smoke directly into his stomach but quickly stopped doing it because of digestive problems. Placing the fingers over the area of the esophagus may detect the movement; in fact, one can momentarily stop the descent of liquid or air by this method. M.C.L. Greene states that such patients can only phonate two or three husky or whispering words at a time after insufflating, and that they whisper most of the time.†

The Soft Palate

Inasmuch as it is necessary to produce compression of air in the mouth and pharynx in order to inject it into the esophagus, the laryngectomee naturally and unconsciously effects and maintains a sealing off of the

---

* He need not worry that the patient will choke; his airway is no longer connected to the feeding pathway. One patient swallowed a handful of sleeping pills at bedtime. He awoke in the morning, but when he swallowed his cup of coffee he collapsed. Since he was up when the medicine took effect, he was quickly pumped out.

† For descriptions of pharyngeal and esophageal action of laryngectomees during speech effort, read Damsté; DiCarlo *et al.*; Diedrich and Youngstrom; Luchsinger and Arnold; Martin 1963; and Snidecor.

nasal pharynx by sharply raising the soft palate (Berg and Moolenaar-Bijl; Damsté; Diedrich and Youngstrom; Snidecor). Patients with palatal insufficiency are unable to generate sufficient intraoral pressure to inject air into the esophagus; they also may have difficulty in producing the plosive consonants which contribute to injection of air. (Berlin 1964). Tests might be made to determine the probability that this can be accomplished. Failure to suck liquids through a straw, to lean forward and suck water from the lip of a cup or from a spoon or to blow up a toy balloon may indicate some weakness in sealing off the nasal pharynx (Damsté; Diedrich and Youngstrom). One need not worry too much about this at the present time because this action may be developed spontaneously when the patient is given compression exercises. However, the speech clinician should be forewarned about any weakness of the palatal function so that he may relate this weakness to the type of responses that the patient makes.

The Tongue

Motility and integrity of the tongue are essential for compressing air and moving it backward into the pharynx and also for accuracy of articulation (Diedrich and Youngstrom). If part of the tongue or underlying tissue has been damaged or resected, or if the nerve endings have been cut, the speech clinician will plan to utilize the remaining or weakened parts for developing and strengthening their function. The usual tests for tongue motility reveal the presence of weakness: rotating the tongue tip around the lip margins; protruding and retracting the tongue; lifting the tongue tip against the alveolar ridge, as for producing /t/, and placing the middle of the tongue against the hard palate, as for producing /k/. Rapid repetition in alternately pronouncing /t/ and /k/ is also useful. The last three functions are particularly essential for the glossal and glossopharyngeal press, that is, for compressing and moving air into the pharynx and esophagus. Regardless of the defects that may be found, we must keep in mind the remarkable adaptation that man applies to overcome physical handicaps. Putney found that some patients so handicapped were able to talk in a limited fashion, saying two or three words per gulp. And we keep recalling the intelligible speech we have heard from a glossectomee!

The Lips

Labile action of the lips and jaw should also be evaluated. The lips must be compressed during one method of injection and must be highly active in the production of plosive consonants, especially in the absence of the pulmonary air stream. Counting in a whisper, using the twenties, thirties, forties, etc., reveals the patient's precision and speed of action, as well as the correct shaping of the lips for the vowels and consonants.

The Jaw

Any weakness of the jaw action is quickly detected by having the patient first lower his jaw during rapid repetition of /wa/, /wa/, /wa/, and second open his mouth markedly for a yawn. (Damsté).

The Teeth

If the speech clinician observes that the patient's dentures are ill-fitting or are completely or partially absent, he must ascertain the latter's plans for correcting the fitting or shortage. Loose-fitting dentures may prevent complete contact of the tongue against the palate for compression (Diedrich and Youngstrom). Likewise, loose-fitting dentures may contribute to poor articulation. One of our club members refused to wear his dentures; saying that they did not fit. As it was, his lips flapped loosely and loudly as he tried to articulate his consonants. He compensated by markedly chopping his jaws. (A dental adhesive is helpful for firming the hold of dentures.) Another patient, who was illiterate, had no teeth and no dentures. His speech with an artificial larynx was unintelligible.

Preoperative Speech

Disregarding the voice quality, which may be impaired by growths, the speech clinician may use the speech and language of a patient as an important diagnostic indication of successful or unsuccessful post-laryngectomy speech. Kallen has commented:

> A not unimportant factor in the prognosis is the patient's manner of speech and articulation before the laryngectomy. Apart from consideration of his age and training, if his speech was clear and well enunciated before the larynx was removed, he is more apt to cultivate a clear and well defined pseudospeech.

The examiner should note, also, the occupation of the person who is speaking so well. The salesman, preacher, politician, labor leader and language teacher all have such a close affinity between spoken language and its associated mental aspects that it is most natural that they will utilize these faculties to reorganize the physical capacities of the revised speech mechanism.

Breathing

The removal of the larynx and separation of pulmonary breathing from the oral-pharyngeal tract does not necessarily mean that defective breathing will not be involved in the production of esophageal speech, M.C.L.

Greene has reported, and we have frequently observed, that laryngectomized persons who, preoperatively, had the habit of clavicular breathing are likely to retain the habit of overtensing the accessory and pharyngeal muscles in the production of alaryngeal speech. We have noticed this phenomenon appear when we use the preinjection "sniff," where the strap muscles bulge, the eyebrows rise and wrinkles appear in the forehead. Such severe tension may prevent easy, relaxed, fluent speech. M.C.L. Greene has pointed out that tense shallow breathers (clavicular breathers) with poor speech prior to laryngectomy may not acquire postoperatively the coordination of respiratory and articulatory muscles that is so necessary for fluency and ease of esophageal speech. It is therefore advisable for the speech clinician to evaluate the effectiveness of each prospective laryngectomee's breathing in the same manner in which laryngeal speakers are examined. M.C.L. Greene even advocates preoperative breathing examinations and subsequent exercises to establish thoracic-diaphragmatic breathing habits that may be coordinated with the newly learned esophageal speech. It would therefore appear very important to evaluate breathing in the preoperative period.

Chapter Six

TEACHING ESOPHAGEAL SPEECH: AN ECLECTIC METHOD

Murphy says that "much of voice therapy is a process of experimentation with the individual's voice." Damsté believes that every laryngectomized person presents a fresh complex of unknown factors which have to be found empirically. Having found the pertinent factors, the therapist must have a "certain amount of mobility" to reach the goal in the shortest possible time. M.C.L. Greene aptly describes the eclectic method:

> The first aim in teaching is the production of a sound; it does not matter how this is achieved, but achieved it must be at the earliest possible moment after the removal of the larynx and for purely psychological reasons. The thing the patient fears most is that he will never again be able to speak. Failure to achieve voice after laryngectomy has the most depressing and disastrous effect upon the patient and may delay speech many months.

Finkbeiner also prefers not to have too rigid a view in teaching laryngectomees because all methods are useful at times but may bring wrong results at any given stage of treatment. M.C.L. Greene applies one principle after another until successful voice is obtained. Berlin (1965a) and Diedrich and Youngstrom state that many good speakers use more than one method of air injection during any given speaking period. Snidecor (1968) advises that once a method has been established, the speaker should be encouraged to experiment with others, unless, in the opinion of the therapist, such experimentation would be confusing. Furthermore, Snidecor (1968) states:

> Within the limitation of the present data, we feel that many esophageal speakers are unconsciously employing a combination of methods of air intake, which we think is commendable

Both M.C.L. Greene and Snidecor (1968) believe that aspiration and injection become "mutually integrated and complementary." Diedrich and Youngstrom's observations showed that patients may use both injection and inhalation in successive syllables. Finally, we must not doggedly continue with speech therapy during many months with a difficult patient who could have been talking with an artificial larynx two or three weeks after he had surgery. Nor should we persist in urging air intake by inhalation

91

on a patient who is aged and debilitated. Such a technique requires a large expenditure of energy and effort during continuous speech. (Snidecor). Likewise, patients with poor supportive breathing or with hearing deficiencies by no means should have imposed on them a single routine of therapy. We have given ample evidence that we should not worry about the method; whatever we begin with may be altered, or replaced, or developed as perceptive progress evolves. Hence, our program of instructions on speech therapy for laryngectomees has been formulated with the purpose of using as many techniques as possible for a specific problem of any given patient. Therefore, we have prepared instructions for teaching different types of air intake, for teaching speech with an artificial larynx and for teaching speech by parallel use of the artificial larynx and esophageal speech.

INSTRUCTIONS FOR TEACHING ESOPHAGEAL SPEECH

The instructions for teaching esophageal speech are an approximation of those that have been used in teaching many patients. They are consistent with the philosophies of contemporary writers as presented in earlier chapters. The instructions are intended to serve as a temporary guide for speech clinicians who wish to become familiar with methods of teaching esophageal speech. As they become more experienced, they can add or substract from these instructions. It is also possible for a laryngectomee to use these instructions to develop his own esophageal speech. We prefer, or rather suggest, that instruction under these conditions should be accompanied by some guidance from a speech clinician or an experienced laryngectomized teacher of esophageal speech.

The left side of each page of instructions contains the information that the instructor gives to the patient. These instructions are always enclosed by quotation marks. The numerals that appear within these instructions refer to the notes located on the right side of the page. Guiding instructions to the speech clinician also appear on the left-hand side of the page but have no quotation marks.

The right side of each page contains numbered instructions that match the numbers on the left side of the page. These instructions refer the clinician to an optional technique, to an explanation for the use of a particular procedure or to a precaution that experience has proved to be important. Lists of words, phrases and sentences also are supplied on the right side. Space is left for the clinician to make notes of any techniques he may have devised and found helpful. A class professor may also suggest a technique which may be written on the right-hand side.

These instructions are designed to be of benefit to all persons who are involved in the laryngectomee's total learning process. The combination of instructions and explanations gives the instructor an understanding of the principles involved in the use of each technique. Since they are also given to the patient, he can more intelligently achieve the desired technique. We find that this feature often aids the patient's perception and speeds his learning.

Because patients often forget or do not understand verbal instructions, it is wise to write practice instructions in duplicate. The patient will have a reminder and the clinician will have a record for future guidance. Many of the techniques used here were inspired by the exchange of ideas between patient and clinician.

The first part of each lesson should be a review of sounds and words that were developed in the previous session. An occasional review of all material used previously is important. The order in which sounds are introduced is entirely optional; the presentation here is made by beginning with the development of unvoiced plosive sounds, which facilitate injection. Other clinicians may wish to use vowels first, especially if they use inhalation for air intake.

Instructions are arranged in short, graduated units. One patient may be able to cover several units in one session, whereas another may take two sessions on a single unit. Since these units take so little time to present, a very alert, energetic patient may be able to accept and learn five or ten units in an hour's session. However, we wish to emphasize the importance of developing accuracy in the early period of instruction as opposed to speed and loudness (Snidecor 1968).

The frequency of lessons depends on the character and the abilities of each patient. Some speech clinicians give one or more lessons (not units) daily, having the patient practice between the sessions. Snidecor urges three lessons on the first day, especially if the patient lives at a distance. This insures successful acquisition of the initial sound before the patient leaves for home. We have found this routine very helpful, both for teaching esophageal speech and for dysphonia of all kinds. The patient may be sent to an adjoining room for practice, if he does not succeed within the first lesson period. He also may return home for practice and return in the afternoon to complete the first series of units. A week of daily lessons or a good start in a three-day period is far more beneficial than ten weeks of weekly lessons. (Note Berlin's report (1963b) on intensive therapy at a Veterans Administration hospital.) The patient does not have time to become discouraged or to shun practice sessions, and mistakes may be corrected before a bad habit has become fixed.

The patient is given the option of using an artificial larynx during the instruction period for esophageal speech. This enables him to talk to the instructor during the lesson period. Both teacher and pupil are relieved from anxiety and delay in communicating with each other.

If he is not using the artificial larynx, the patient should abandon the writing pad as soon as he can say a few words and phrases, no matter how slow they may be. The wiser criterion is the attainment by the patient of a positive confidence that he can communicate somewhat intelligibly with what vocabulary he has. Of course, he can always communicate with an artificial larynx. Under such circumstances, then, the time may come when he may be urged to abandon the instrument, too. The speech clinician can further the development of the patient's vocabulary by obtaining from him the common phrases and vocabulary used in his work.

Periodic Tests for measuring the patient's improvement in esophageal speech are found below. These tests should show the patient the progress he is making in relearning to talk and should encourage him to continue with therapy until he has acquired a satisfactory voice.

Various manuals for teaching esophageal speech are listed in the Appendix. We urge both teachers and laryngectomees to become familiar with the numerous techniques found in them. They are also an excellent source for words and phrases that can supplement the words used here.

PERIODIC TESTS FOR MEASURING IMPROVEMENT IN SPEECH

Tests have been prepared to enable the laryngectomee to "visualize his progress" (Wepman *et al.*) and to stimulate him to continue to improve his speech instead of withdrawing from instruction. The tests should be given periodically as indicated in the lesson section. Test results and dates are recorded on each test form. The patient should be cautioned that he need not worry about the early test results; rather, the goal is to show him how much he improves from the beginning of instruction.

Test 1. Phonating *ah* and *pah* on Demand

Ask the patient to say *ah*. After five seconds, ask him to say it again. Do not rush him. Continue until he has made ten attempts. The criterion for a successful completion is a recognizable vowel. Indicate the number of successful completions in ten attempts. Failure is indicated if he fails to make a sound in five seconds.

Test 2. Time Interval Required for Initiation of an Esophageal Sound

Signal the speaker to say *ah*, starting a stopwatch and stopping it when the speaker says the word. You may also watch the second hand of a wristwatch. The test is repeated five times, first with *ah* and second with *pah*. Average the times required for each sound and record them on the test form with the date.

Test 3. Prolonging a Vowel: Isolated and with an Initial Consonant

Instruction to speaker: "Let's find how long you can hold a sound like *ah* (or *pah*). When I say *ah*, repeat it and hold it as long as you can without taking in more air. Get ready: say *ah*."

To the speech clinician: Record the time from a stopwatch or wristwatch from the moment the sound is heard to the instant it ceases. Do the same with the syllable *pah*. Repeat each test five times and record the average for each syllable and the date on the test form.

Test 4. Repeating Syllables on One Air Intake Without Pause, Using *ah* and *pah*

Instruction to speaker: "Let's see how many times you can repeat *ah* on one air intake. When I say 'go,' take in air and keep saying *ah, ah, ah* as long as you can. Ready? Go!"

To the speech clinician: Do the same test with *pah*. Count the number of syllables spoken on five attempts, average the results and record with the date. If the patient endeavors to inject in the middle of the repetition, count only the syllables produced up to that moment. Caution: count only one syllable for a prolonged *ah* or *pah*.

Test 5. Counting as Many Numbers as Possible in One Air Intake

Instruction to speaker: "Will you take in air and count from one up as long as you can? Stop when you can't say a number or if you try to inject air again. Say each number clearly. Start when I say 'Go!' Ready? Go!"

To the speech clinician: If the patient injects during the count, record only the numbers spoken up to the moment of the second injection. Then remind the patient that he did it, and tell him to avoid doing it on the next attempt. Repeat each test five times and record the averages and date on the record form.

Test 6. Time Interval and Air Intake While Reading a Plosive-Laden Sentence and a Sentence Without Plosives (Sixteen Syllables)

Instruction to speaker: "Will you please read this sentence? When I say 'Go,' start reading. Ready? Go!"

To the speech clinician: Start the stopwatch when the patient produces the first speech sound and stop it when the last sound is heard. At the same time, mark down the number of injections made during the reading. Repeat the test five times for each sentence and average the time intervals and the number of air intakes. If research is intended on a large number of patients, the two sentences should be alternated with every other patient.

1. *Jack's riding downtown tonight at six o'clock to get two spring suits.*
2. *If you have aluminumware in your home, you may live longer.*

Test 7. Speed of Reading a Prose Passage

Instruction to speaker: "Will you start reading this paragraph in a natural easy manner? Do not read the numbers that appear between the lines. They are for counting the number of words read. You will read for sixty seconds. When I say 'Go.' start reading. Stop when I say 'Stop.' Ready? Go!"

To the speech clinician: First have the patient read the paragraph in silence. Then have him read it aloud for one minute. Count the number of words that he read. Repeat the reading five times and average the number of words. Record the results and date on the record form.

When the sunlight strikes raindrops in the air, they act [10] like a prism and form a rainbow. The rainbow is [20] a division of white light into many beautiful colors. These [30] take the shape of a long round arch, with its [40] path high above, and its two ends apparently beyond the [50] horizon. There is, according to legend, a boiling pot of [60] gold at one end. People look, but no one ever [70] finds it. When a man looks for something beyond his [80] reach, his friends say he is looking for the pot [90] of gold at the end of the rainbow.

Throughout the [100] centuries men have explained the rainbow in various ways. Some [110] have accepted it as a miracle without physical explanation. To [120] the Hebrews it was a token that there would be [130] no more universal floods. The Greeks used to imagine that [140] it was a sign from the gods to foretell war [150] or heavy rain.

Periodic Test Results

Test 1. Phonating *ah* and *pah* on demand

No. of Successes

Dates	ah	pah

Criteria of success: Berlin's good speakers made twenty successful attempts on command after fourteen lesson-days. Poor speakers took twenty-four days. These are not suitable criteria because the training was condensed. You will get some criteria by testing your own patients.

Test 2. Time Interval Required for Initiation of an Esophageal Sound

Time Intervals

Dates	ah	pah

Criteria of success: Good speakers inject in only $\frac{1}{2}$ second and speak about $\frac{1}{5}$ second later (Diedrich and Youngstrom). A time interval of one second may be used for comparison purposes. Average the five attempts for each sound and record.

Test 3. Prolonging a Vowel: Isolated and with an Initial Consonant

No. of Seconds

Dates	ah	pah

Criteria of success: Average duration for *ah* is 2.3 seconds (Berlin 1965b). No record is available for prolonging a vowel reinforced with a plosive consonant. Average the five attempts for each sound and record.

Test 4. Repeating Syllables on One Air Intake Without Pause, Using *ah* and *pah*

No. of Syllables

Dates   ah   pah

Criteria for success: The average of syllables per air-charge for *ah* is ten for very good speakers, eight for adequate speakers and four for poor speakers. (Berlin 1965a). There is no record for *pah*. Average the number of syllables for *ah* and *pah* and record.

Test 5. Counting as Many Numbers as Possible in One Air Intake

No. of Digits

Dates   ah   pah

Criteria for success: Snidecor's six patients averaged eight digits with a range of 4 to 10 (1968). Average the number of digits for five attempts and record. *Note:* The number 7 has two syllables, which would mean one more syllable than there are digits.

Test 6. Time Interval and Air Intakes While Reading a Plosive-Laden Sentence and a Sentence Without Plosives

No. of Seconds

Dates   Plosive   Nonplosive

Criteria for success: The plosive-laden sentence should be shorter than the nonplosive-laden sentence. Average the five attempts in seconds for each sentence and record.

Test 7. Speed of Reading a Prose Passage

Dates   Words per Minute

Criteria for success: Sixty words per minute is adequate for patients who have just finished their training period. Snidecor's six good speakers averaged 113 words per minute with a range of 85 to 129. Average the number of words read for one minute during five attempts and record.

SEVEN PHASES OF TEACHING ESOPHAGEAL SPEECH

Phase I. Orientation and Preliminary Testing

Unit 1. Gratitude and Expectations

To the speech clinician: This introductory talk may be altered according to your wishes. We have found it very informative and it makes a favorable impression on the patient.

"I am sure you have a fairly good idea whether you are going to talk again.[1] Your surgeon has done a good job of clearing up the disease; the nurses have been wonderful in caring for and feeding you, and the club visitors have given you living proof that laryngectomees do talk again. When we come right down to reality, you have not lost as much as you might think. Rather, you have much to be thankful for. You can hear and see; you can eat and drink; you can read and write; you can walk, run and drive a car. You have your family and friends; you can do about everything you did except swim, and some people do that. You have most of your speech mechanism: your mouth, lips, teeth and tongue. You can smile. You breathe more easily than normal speakers.[2] Your chief loss is the sound maker, your larynx or vibrator. Your voice maker is gone but thousands of people have found that the surgeons have left a different kind of voice box or vibrator at about the same place in the throat. So laryngectomees can 'Thank God that He gave them two voices in a single lifetime.' "[3]

Unit 2. Demonstrating the Artificial Larynx

"Perhaps I should say that we have three voices, because there is a third way you can talk, and you can learn it in about three minutes. I am showing this to you in order to assure you that you will always be able to talk by one

[1] It is helpful to have the patient's spouse at the first session so that both persons know the techniques. We have often trained the wife to produce an esophageal sound in order to help the patient. Even the children have fun using it!

[2] V.F. Pekarek, M.D., a laryngectomee, states that the laryngectomee breathes with less resistance than the normal person.

[3] This sentence was first spoken by Paul W. Augenstein, Marion, Ohio, at a meeting of the Cleveland Lost Chord Club. It is the motto on the club's monthly bulletin.

way or another.[1] This is an artificial larynx.[2] On this end is a vibrating diaphragm. When I place it against my neck, the sound comes out of my mouth. I will whisper *one-two-three*.[3] ... You heard no sound. Next, I will press the button to start the vibrator as I whisper *one-two-three*. ... That's the voice you can use to talk. Try it yourself. First count with your lips and tongue while I hold the vibrator on your neck without pressing the button. . . . You made no sound.[4] Now whisper again while I press the button as you say *one-two three*. ... Good. Do it again. ... Say *hello*. ... Say *how are you?* ... You are talking again! With this aid some people go to work right after they are well. Many laryngectomees don't like the sound, so they won't use it; others discard it as soon as they are able to talk again. So you don't need to worry about not being able to talk. You have proved to yourself that you can. You can talk to your friends over the telephone tomorrow, or you can use it in your business."[5]

[1] The Bell Telephone Electronic Larynyx is used here as a sample demonstration. Other models may be used and described, such as Aurex and Kett-Mark models. The ones with the tube in the mouth would require a longer learning time at this point.

[2] If you have already shown the artificial larynx in the preoperative interview, you may wish to change the instruction accordingly.

[3] Throughout the therapy in this book, ellipses will be used to indicate that you or the patient have spoken.

[4] Be sure the diaphragm is held snugly against the neck; otherwise, free noise will mask the spoken sounds. If the patient has had x-ray treatments that thickened the tissues, he should use the Cooper-Rand model with the tube in his mouth.

[5] At this point, you must ask the patient to decide what he wishes to do: use the instrument to talk with while he is learning esophageal speech, use it exclusively or use it with parallel instruction. Be sure he understands the advantages of each combination.

Unit 3. Probing for Esophageal Speech Sounds

"People all over the world talk with this kind of appliance but you should know something much more important. People talk in many languages which contain over 375 different kinds of speech sounds.[1] That is how adaptable man is; he can go to a new country and learn an entirely different language, but it is spoken

[1] Judson and Weaver.

with the same kind of a speech mechanism. Men of all nations have to learn to speak again when they lose the larynx. They use their speech mechanisms to talk in a slightly different manner.

"Let's hear what sounds you may be able to make at this time.[2] Perhaps you have already discovered that you can make a speech sound. Do you recall after you had eaten a meal at the hospital, you were surprised to hear a sound deep in your throat as you tried to talk? . . . When you were a youngster, did you belch after eating a big meal of chicken, cake and watermelon at a picnic? ... No? Well, I'll make a burp. ... You try one. ... You can't do it? . . . Just swallow some air and burp it back up. ... No success![3] Don't worry. Others don't do it at first and still others don't like to do it.

"The speech sound that we use is not really a burp. In fact, laryngectomees make sounds in different ways. Here is one way they make it. I'll say *pah*. That had a sound that came from the throat but it wasn't a real burp, and the /p/ sound was made in the mouth. We call such consonants *plosives* because they are made by exploding compressed air. Let's hear you make a /p/ sound. ... Just pop it out between your lips. ... Try once more. ... That's almost right. Say it once more and tell me if you hear yourself make the /p/. ...[4] You heard it? ... That's good. Then, let's work on it. Say something with it; say *pah*. ... You whispered it. Say it with voice. ... Sometimes it comes without thinking. Once more, say *pah*. ...[5]

"Let's try another sound. Say /t/. ... Good. Say /k/. ... Watch me make it. ... You make it. ... That's it; say it with *kah;* full voice. ... You whispered it. Say it with voice. ... Try to make a hiss. ... Say *saw*. ... Try this sound: chop. ... Try *stop*. ...[6]

"We've tried a burp and a plosive sound to

[2] You may already have heard the patient make a burp when he whispered in the hospital.

[3] Make notes of the patient's success in making the preliminary esophageal sounds.

[4] If the patient does not hear the voiceless /p/, give him the amplified sound by earphones or use TOK-BAK (See Appendix). You may already have tested his hearing and are forewarned.

[5] Record success or failure.

[6] Record success or failure.

get air out of the throat. Let's try a third one. Do you know how to pant? ... Breathe in and out like a dog does on a hot day. ... Good. Now instead of just breathing in air into your lungs, breathe into your throat, then say *ah*. ... Make a sharp sniff with your nose; feel the air go down. ...[7] Did you feel air going into your throat? ... No? Try it once more; sniff sharply through your nose. ... Well, let's make a final try. Sniff sharply and say *ah*. ...[8] Now, we are going to start over with one of the other methods of making an esophageal sound."

To the speech clinician: At this point, give Periodic Test 1 (page 97).

[7] If the patient shows a basic skill in injecting air, the method he used may be the first method in the formal effort to obtain the esophageal sound.

[8] Record success or failure.

Unit 4. Speech Clinician's Talk to the Wife of a Laryngectomee

To the speech clinician: This sample talk may be given to the wife of the laryngectomee after the preliminary testing of the patient, or while the patient is practicing attempts to produce an esophageal sound in an adjoining room, or by special appointment.

"Mrs. Jones, I want to thank you for coming in so that you can become acquainted with some of the problems that your husband will be having while he is learning to talk. Your attitude and cooperation will be most valuable, helpful and necessary to insure success for your husband. In other words, you have an important part in the program. I wish to make some explanations that will help you to understand what we are doing and what you can do. You are always welcome to sit in on part of the instruction period. I may ask you to do this from time to time to keep informed of how you can help your husband.

"1. The first thing to remember is that you must not expect too much improvement in your husband's speech at first. It may take him longer than others to learn to take in air and use it for speech. But he may come along faster than others. Be patient about his progress.

"2. The next point is to watch your husband's lips while he tries to talk. Never get discouraged and look away; that will discourage him and prove that he is failing to communicate. Watching lips may help you to understand enough to know what he is saying. But don't move your own lips; he will think you are not understanding him! Stop doing something which requires looking down at your work, such as sewing, and watch his face. Listen to him talk without turning your eyes or head. He will require time to give you information, so it demands your attention and patience.

"3. Always encourage your husband in every way and give him the impression that you expect him to learn to talk. If he does not practice, gently urge him to do so. He may get angry at you for bossing him, but he must be reminded that doing things thousands of times is necessary to learn esophageal speech.

"4. Don't wait too long for him to get an idea across to you. It is better to offer him the magic slate or scratch pad than for both of you to be frustrated and discouraged. [Likewise, the artificial larynx may be used to avoid embarrassment.]

"5. Invite his friends to come to see him; insist that he go out with you. Eventually you will want to send him to the store for some groceries. Let him go alone; he will enjoy the feeling that he is able to do the same things he did before. He may succeed in talking to someone.

"6. By all means, make arrangements for him to attend the Lost Chord Club Meetings, and be sure to go with him. Let it be taken for granted that he will go.

"7. If any trouble comes up, always call me or one of the wives of the club. The surgeon is always ready to help you. Here is an emergency card which contains the telephone numbers of some of the wives. Don't hesitate to call upon them at any time."

Phase II. Initiating the Esophageal Speech Sound

Units 5 through 15 comprise the techniques that are used to initiate the esophageal speech sound by all available methods. The patient receives instruction that gives him understanding and experience first in compressing air within the mouth, then in compressing and injecting it into the esophagus. The assistance of the voiceless plosive consonants in compressing and injecting is added to the earlier techniques. The patient is next shown how to use the peculiar action of /s/ in injecting part of its compressed air into the esophagus. After acquiring or attempting to acquire the above skills, the patient is trained in compressing and injecting air by the piston action of the tongue. The unique feature of this system is that the patient can acquire increasingly effective skills in compressing and injecting air. However, if he does not succeed up to this point, the patient may be trained in the method of inhaling air into the esophagus.

Whenever the patient first acquires good injection at any point in the progressive units, he must return to the first step, Unit 5, in order to add the effective action of plosive consonants to his skill at compressing and injecting, or at inhaling air into the esophagus. He thus always obtains training in skills covered by Units 5 to 15. Along with others (Damsté; Diedrich and Youngstrom; Moolenaar-Bijl 1953a; Snidecor; Stetson 1937a), we have found that once the patient can make an esophageal sound by any method, progress toward fluency may be more rapidly attained with the plosive consonant action. This is especially true of those who first learn the inhalation method of air intake. They can do the vowels fairly well but are slow in acquiring skill at producing consonants. Even Hodson and Oswald, strong advocates of inhalation, start their patients with /k/ and /g/. Hence, we feel it advisable to move to plosive sounds as soon as the patient develops an esophageal sound.

If the patient does not acquire esophageal sound by being exposed to the numerous methods found in Phase II, the clinician should simply start all over from the beginning until he succeeds by one method or another. Nothing is lost by trying two or more methods in succession on the patient because the patient gains additional experience and insight from manipulating his speech parts to compress and inject air. We have had patients who could not do this after repeated attempts. We then sent them into an adjoining room to practice at their leisure. They became relieved of tension and anxiety and had time calmly to review and try out the techniques presented to them. The patients were usually successful upon their return to the therapist, but if they still required further effort, they were permitted to go back to the motel to practice at frequent in-

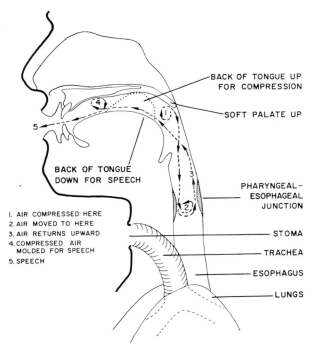

Figure 12. Postlaryngectomy speech mechanism. (*Courtesy of American Medical Association*)

tervals and return the next morning. It is rare to have a failure under such circumstances unless there are positive signs of inability to produce the desired sounds. Then the therapist should reexamine the case history and perhaps consult with the surgeon to ascertain possible causes for failure to obtain esophageal voice.

It would appear that we have set up a formidable chore to offer a new patient (Units 5 to 15) on his first formal visit for speech instruction. However, the experience of clinicians shows that the instruction moves rapidly from unit to unit. Furthermore, we do not insist that the clinician follow our sequence of stimulating the patient for the first esophageal sound. His experience may be different from ours. It is always wise to change to another method if a patient does not acquire esophageal sound by one technique. Flexibility in instruction methods always should be maintained because of the variations in personality of both patient and clinician.

Unit 5. Relaxation and Breathing

"Here is an outline of your throat the way it is now (Fig. 12).[1] The larynx was removed, leaving one passage for food, which passes from your mouth and throat into the esophagus. You breathe in and out through the stoma, the opening in your neck. The area where your larynx was is now slightly narrowed so that the esophagus becomes a vibrator for your new voice. This vibrator has to have air forced into its opening before it can make a voiced sound. The mouth of the vibrator ordinarily opens only when food comes down to be swallowed. For voice, you must open it to move air in and then vibrate the air as it comes out.

"The easiest way to open the esophagus is to stay relaxed. You never need to strain or work hard to get the sound in or out for esophageal speech. Let me show you what I mean by strain or tension and its opposite, relaxation. Double up your fist and keep clenching it as hard as you can. That's the extreme of tension. Now open it and let the muscles go. Feel how different it is. That's what I mean by relaxation. Here's another way to show it. Rest your hand on my index finger. Let its weight be on my finger. Watch what happens when I remove

[1] This explanation and Figure 12 may be used as an introduction and orientation of the patient to the physiology of air intake. Some speech clinicians believe that explanations confuse the patient. Hence, you must use your own judgment in this matter. We found it to be very helpful to the patient's understanding.

my finger. ... Your hand hung up there without
support. That means your muscles were
naturally tensed for holding up the arm. This
time, let out all of the strength from your muscles. Have support only from my finger. Let
your muscles go! Let the arm rest loosely. ...
Your hand dropped quickly when I withdrew
my finger. You had relaxed some of your muscles. That's what I mean by relaxing. Your neck
and throat muscles must not be tight; otherwise, they will interfere with an easy phonation.

"Let's try to become relaxed through breathing and sighing.[2] Inhale slowly and sigh. ...
Don't blow out the air. Breathe in and let it
flow out gently. ... Good. Also, nod your head
backward as you inhale and let it fall forward
of its own weight.[3] ... That's better. Let's do
it five times, easy in and easy out. Let your
head drop forward as if you had no muscles. ...
Feel how easy your neck muscles are. There is
no tension, and that is the way it should be
when we try to take in air and use it for speech.
Remember, you don't use your neck muscles
to talk. If you become anxious or try hard to
talk, you can't do it well."[4]

Unit 6. Demonstration of Compression

"Now, we are ready to try some methods of
getting air into your esophagus. Several methods are available. Here's one way. You use the
lips and cheeks to explode the air backward.
Puff up your cheeks with air and keep your
lips tightly closed. ... You've trapped a ball of
air in your mouth. We have to move that air
into your throat and esophagus. I will press my
hands against your cheeks but don't let air escape through your lips. I'll say 'Now' when I
press. Now! ... You let the lips pop open. Keep
them firmly closed so you can feel what
happens to the air. Again, Now! ... What happened to the air? ... You felt some of it go back
into your throat. Once more, feel a fullness in

[2] Read M.C.L. Greene's description of relaxation to ease
the tension in the area of
the neck.

[3] Stand beside the patient and
gently push the head forward
to show the patient how to
let it go.

[4] Give the patient frequent
rests in all exercises, during
which explanations may be
given.

your throat as the air goes down. Now! ... You got a little fullness. Once again. Puff up your cheeks; Now! ... You felt the air go down that time![1] I'll do it once more so you can get a definite feeling of air moving into your throat. Now! ... You felt it? ... Good. See what you can do by yourself. Simply puff up your cheeks and push them in sharply. Don't let air escape through your lips. ... Did you move air into the throat? ... Not yet.[2] It happens more easily if you open up your throat like a yawn. Open up your throat, press your cheeks and move the air backward into the throat. ... Do it differently this time. Compress your cheeks and lips without pushing in on the cheeks and at the same time drop the back of the tongue. .. You felt air move but not into the throat. Try it again. ... You felt it go into your throat? ... Good. That's what we have to do before we can send the air back up to make speech sounds."

[1] A mouth full of water is more effective and dramatic, but it requires a plastic sheet to protect the patient's clothing. Also, you must stand away from the patient's lips in case he lets the water squirt out by chance. The patient is sure to feel the water move down, which demonstrates movement.

[2] If the patient doesn't feel the air entering the esophagus, you might tell him to swallow as you press the cheeks. Ordinarily we do not use that expression because of the danger of establishing a wrong impression or habit, but it is necessary in some situations.

Unit 7. Injection Aided by Voiceless Plosive Consonants

"Let's try another way to move air.[1] A moment ago I asked you to keep your lips tightly closed. Now, I am asking you to open your lips to make the sound /p/. When you say that sound, you can only do it by compressing some air first and then exploding it through your lips. Some of the air is used to produce the explosion but some of it also is forced backward into the throat. That air may help you to make the vowel in *pah*. First, let's make the sound /p/. ... Good. Repeat /p/ five times very fast and feel some air moving into the throat.[2] ... You did feel some air moving? ... Good. Try it again.[3] ... We are going to do something with that air. Say /p/ four times very fast and sharply and when you feel that some air has moved into your throat, say *pah*. ... That was a good try. Do it again and try to come out with a clear audible *pah*. ... I heard something, a soft sound. Did you hear it? ... Did you feel the

[1] Always talk in a manner that conveys the impression that you are relaxed.

[2] Use the familiar popping of air against a piece of paper to demonstrate lip action and the force of the explosion.

[3] Blowing through a straw into water helps to develop compression. Blow up a rubber balloon with an air pump, then release the air between the closed lips of the patient. He feels the air rush back.

pressure down there? ... Once more, keep your throat open as we told you before and say four /p/ sounds and then get a good *pah*. ... I heard it again. That is what we call air injection. You compress air, move it back into the throat and then say a word like *pah*.

"Next, we are going to exaggerate that action. Open your mouth wide and snap it shut with your lips closing tightly the way a fish takes water into its mouth. Do it rapidly four times and feel the air flowing into your throat. ... You got more air than you did before. Do the fish mouth four times and quickly say *pah*.[4] ... Don't pause a moment. Get it in and out fast. Once more.[5] ... That's better. I heard a vowel. Once more, end with a clear *pah*. ... That was very definitely a voiced sound. Do it again before you forget how you did it. ... Did you hear it? Did you feel how it was done? ... Good. That's your new voice![6]

"We first tried to get you to move the air spontaneously by using the plosive sound /p/. Next, we want you to make a more deliberate conscious effort to move the air backward. As you pronounce /p/ say it backward; that is, squeeze all of the air backward and downward instead of exploding it forward between your lips.[7] You will still make an audible /p/ sound with the action. Relax your throat to admit the air into the esophagus.

"Let's try it. Send the air backward as you say /p/. ... That was about right. Once more; deliberately use your cheeks, lips and tongue to squeeze the air back. ... You got a good /p/ but did you feel the air go down? ... Good. You can use that air to say *ah*. Force all of the air down and then say /pɑh/. Now you know you can inject air into your esophagus. Practice doing it many times at home."

Unit 8. Using the Voiceless Consonant /t/

"Let's try another sound. When I say /t/, I place the tongue against and behind my upper

[4] The whistle technique is also helpful. If the patient can make a sharp whistle with it, he has a correct tongue movement for compression. (See page 156.)

[5] Snidecor; and Berlin 1965a emphasize the importance of getting the air in fast and the sound out fast. It should take less than one second. Fluency cannot be attained without enough speed to make the two actions occur as one unit.

[6] If you do not have success with /p/, go right into working with /t/. Continue until you have success and then return to Unit 6 and move through the units again.

[7] Forcing water from the mouth into the esophagus is similar to the required injection of air during the production of /p/. Instead of exploding all of the air outward through the lips, Snidecor (1968, p. 163) instructs the patient deliberately to move the air backward and downward into the esophagus, provided he relaxes the latter.

front teeth. I build up pressure behind it and drop the tongue quickly to explode the /t/. You must compress air to make the sound heard. Say /t/ five times. ... That was good action but did you hear it? Make the /t/ loud enough to hear it. ... Did you feel that compressed air helped you to make the /t/? ... Good, that's what we mean by compression. You must build pressure in your mouth because you don't have any air from the lungs to help you. The tongue does the work; you don't have to strain a muscle to do it. Here's more compression. Say /p/ first and then /t/. ... Good! Let's use that pressure. Say /p/, /t/ four times fast[1] and then say *tah*. ... You're coming. You'll get voice this time. Do four fast sounds of /t/ and then say *tah*. ... Good. Say /t/ just twice and follow with *tah*. ... Say /t/ and then *tah*. ... Now say *tah*. ... That's it. Can you do that *pah* again? ... How about *tah*? ... That means you can do some one-syllable words.

"You should be able to say these words. We'll record them on tape and play them back. Try this: *pat*. ... Whenever you have trouble getting started talking, always think of saying /p/; it will get you started. Say /p/, /p/, *pat*.[2] ... That's another word, Say *pot*. ... How about *pop*? ... Say *tah*. ... Now *tot*. ... Let's try some vowels with /t/ and /p/. Say *pay*. ... *pie*. ... *pea*. ... *poo*. We can say a lot of words with /p/, /t/ and the vowels.[3] Try *pat*. ... *tie*. ... *top*. ... *two*. ... Good. Take these words and practice them in the next room.[4] Before you go let's play the words you have used. ... You had better practice making good sharp plosives; that will give you a better chance of producing the vowels."

Unit 9. The Voiceless Plosive Consonant /k/

"How did you get along with those words? Let's hear some of them. Say *pah*. ... Now *tah*. ... That wasn't very clear. Once more. ... Better. Build up pressure behind the tongue and explode the /t/. ... Good. Now say *pah, tah*. Say

---

[1] These are voiceless sounds (not voiced) but they develop some pressure, which is their characteristic.

[2] A comma between sound units, syllables or words means that a definite pause is made between them. A dash between units, syllables or words means that a continuous phonation should be made of those units. This arrangement will be carried out throughout the text.

[3] Have the patient practice the words:

pie; pay; pat; pet; put; pot; papa; pit; pop; pip; two; pep; toe; tie; tight; tote; tape; tap; tea; top; tate; teet; tight; tote; toot; tape; pet; type; tope; tout; taught; pout; toy; pay; pea; pie; poe; poo.

[4] This procedure varies with the patient; some will not be ready for practice with words, but will need more instruction on compression. Continue with /k/, etc., until success is attained as explained earlier.

pay. ... pea, pie, poe, poo. ... You got good explosion on all of them. Practice those words hundreds of times at home.

"Here is a third plosive sound, /k/. This will give you more experience in building up pressure in your mouth and throat. We will put /k/ on the ends of words first because it is easier to say it there.[1] Try the word *take.* ... Make the /k/ like you always did. You have to build up some pressure back of the tongue to get a good, clear /k/. Try *take* once more. ... That's better. Say *took.* ... *tuck.* ... *take-it.* ... The /k/ is really pronounced with the *it,* so it sounds like *ta-kit.* Try it. ... Good; that was two syllables! Next, we'll put the /k/ at the beginning of a word, but we'll sneak up on it this way: *ta-kit.* ... Again, *ta-kit.* ... Then *kit.* ... Good. Hear and feel it! Say *kit.* ... Now you can say *cat.* ... *cup.* ... *cape.* ... *cook.* ... *cot.* .. *kitty.* ... That came out easily.

"You have been making the /k/ sound without knowing exactly how important it is for compressing air into the esophagus.[2] So let's do five /k/ sounds real fast, one after the other. ... Good. Did you feel the air moving into your throat? ... Good. You are beginning to understand what is needed to get air moving into the throat. Let's say *kay.* ... *kee.* ... *kie.* ... *koe.* ... *koo.* ... You did these faster than you did the previous words. Perhaps you can do two syllables together. Let's experiment. Say *kay-kee.* ... *kie-koe.* ... Good. Say *kitty.* ... *bake-it.* ... *back-up.* ... *pick-up.* ... Here's a chance for you to say a word you use every day. Say *OK.* ... You haven't worked on initial vowels yet, so we will first try *kokay.* Now, say *kokay.* Say it this way with a very short rest between the two words: *kokay, OK.* ... Better do it this way: say both of them with one effort or phonation: *kokay-OK.* ... You got it easily that time. Of course, you should not say *OK* that way; just think of saying the /k/ but don't say it. Some

[1] Snidecor states that the final sound is easier to say than the initial consonant.

[2] Not all patients move this fast. The important point is that you are helping them to build up pressure in different ways. If no results are obtained, don't be discouraged. Explain that you have many techniques to use. Then proceed with the following units according to our plan. By the time the patient has been put through the units once or twice he will have developed esophageal sound action. If not, other procedures are available.

people actually rehearse the /k/ unnoticed by the auditor.[3] They slightly protrude their lips but it is enough to inject some air into the esophagus. So start saying *OK* to your family. Here's a list of words that have /k/ at the end or at the beginning.[4] Remember, if you have trouble with initial /k/, say a word first that has /k/ at the end; like *take-kate*. Do those on one air-charge, that is, without pausing."

[3] Moolenaar-Bijl   (1953b) mentions this incipient use of a plosive to initiate a vowel. More about vowels later on.

[4] Have the patient say these words hundreds of times:

pick; tick; tock; take; tack; poke; pack; tack; key; cup; cat; coop; coot; coat; cop; kid; kiddy; caw; cake; kick; cock; kill; kilt; coy; call; tuck; teak; took; puck; poke; tick-tock; kitty; kitty-cat; tic-tac; tic-tac-toe; pick-it; skip-it; keep-it; tack-it; take-it; tuck-it.

The two-syllable combinations are offered here only because some patients will be ready for them, and they are excellent practice material. Two-syllable words will be given formally in Unit 16.

Unit 10. Adding the Sound /s/ to the Injection Action

"How did you get along with the /k/ words?[1] ... Let's hear you say /k/ with the five vowels. ... Good. and how about *OK*? ... Good! Did you try it on your wife and friends? ... Fine. How about greeting a person with *Hi*? Try that. ... You have trouble with the vowels at present. You can't say the /h/ anyway, so just say the vowel. They will understand. You might try saying *kie*, making a very soft /k/. Try it ... That's the idea. Practice on it so you can greet your friends with it.

"You have done well with three consonants, /p/, /t/ and /k/. Now we'll start with the /s/ sound. This will give you still more help in getting air into the esophagus. When you say /s/, part of the air pressure is used to produce the sound and the other part is forced into the esophagus. That helps you with the sounds that follow the /s/. Can you make a hissing sound?

[1] This beginning review is dependent on whether the patient returns at this time from a practice period in a room or at home.

... No, don't blow from the stoma; that doesn't help. You concentrate and compress air behind the tip of the tongue and hiss it out over the tip. Try once more; make a hiss. ... Do it another way. First say /t/ and then follow with /s/, like this: /ts/, as in *its*.[2] Say /ts/ five times and stretch out the /s/ sound. ... Well, let's say some words that end with /s/. Say *kiss*. ... Hold the final /s/ several seconds, if you can. ... That's coming. Say *cuss*. ... Now say *pets*. ... *cats*. ... *cuts*. ... You're getting a good /s/. The /t/ helped you get more air pressure. Try this word: *pussy*. ... Stretch out the vowel at the end and make it *pusseeee*. ... You said *see* at the end. Try it again all in one air-charge. ... You ended again with *see*. Do it this way: *pussee, see*.[3] Do it with two words: *see, see*. ... That's good enough for you to try some vowels with /s/. Say *pussee, say*. ... *pussee, see*. ... *pusseee, sigh*. ... *pussee, so*. ... *pussee, soo*. ... Now repeat them without the *pussee*. ... A moment ago you couldn't do an initial /s/. You are learning fast. Let's work on the final /s/. People often fail to sound it clearly. Say *kits*. ... *pits*. ... *coats*. ... *pats*. ...

Let's blend some more /s/ words from *pussee*. Say *pussee-sit, sit*.[4] ... *pussee-suit, suit*. ... *pussee-soap, soap*. ... Let's try a new combination: say *sip-soup*. ... *soap-sap*. ... *sip-sup*. ... Here are some blends of consonants with /s/. Say *spay*. ... *spee*. ... *spy*. ... *spoe*. ... *spoo*. ... Try *stay*. ... *stee*. ... *stye*. ... *stow*. ... *stew*. ... Also *skay*. ... *skee*. ... *sky*. ... *skoe*. ... *skoo*. ... Practice on this list of words."[5]

[2] Another method of getting the /s/ sound is to reverse the order of /s/ and /t/ as in *pets*. The /t/ action arrests the flow of air from /s/ and builds up pressure that will move air backward. Some patients start at once when asked to say *stop, stay*, etc., after experiencing the production of /s/. See McClear (1960).

[3] This two-word combination is helpful in getting a good attack on the initial sound. The first word ends with *see* followed by a silent pause and an attempt to say *see* without the blend. This will be used throughout the text.

[4] This trio of words will be used throughout the text to develop carryover from the newly developed word. The dash indicates that the two connected words are done with one air-charge, if possible, then there is a pause before the final word.

[5] The patient should practice these words for /s/ hundreds of times:

say; see; sigh; sow; soo; sit; sat; seat; sup; sip; siss; puss; soup; sop; soap; side; supper; saw; seat; seep; step; stop; stick; stack; sky; stuck; spook; speak; spoke; scat; cups; hops; peeps; takes; task; spay; spee; spy; spoe; spoo; skay; skee; sky; skoe; skoo; stay; stee; stye; stow; stew; sop-it; tisket; tasket; set-it; set-it-up; stop-it; stop-it-up; scoop it; scoop-it-up; spit-it-out; speak-it; toy-set.

Unit 11. More Sounds with /s/: /ʃ/ (*sh*) and /tʃ/ (*ch*)

"Two more consonants that have the s-factor as a component are /ʃ/ (*sh*) and /tʃ/ (*ch*). Let's try the /ʃ/ sound first. You lift your tongue slightly more than you do for making /s/, and protrude your lips slightly. First say *kiss*. ... Hold the /s/ longer and glide to the *sh*, like this: *kissssh*, by lifting your tongue tip slightly after you start the /s/. Try it again; get a good lip protrusion for *sh*. ... Good. Now say *kiss-cash*. ... *puss-push*. ... *bus-bush*. ... *tuss-tush*. ... Say *cash-sash*, *she*. ... *cash-shell*, *shell*. ... *ship-shape*, *shape*. ... *sash-shop*, *shop*. ... *sea-shell*. ... *she-shell*. ... Take this list for practice.[1] Repeat the words many times.

"Let's try the /tʃ/ sound. Put the tongue behind the upper front teeth as for /t/ and combine it with the *sh* as in *she* and say the two sounds as one. Try this: *cash-catch*. ... *hash-hatch*. ... *hiss-hitch*. ... Say *ch* five times rapidly, then say *chew*. ... Now say *catch-chew*. ... *catch-chew*, *chew*. ... *catch-chop*, *chop*. ... *teach-cheese*, *cheese*. ... *catch-chair*, *chair*. ... Let's try some single words: *change*. ... *choice*. ... *chuck*. ... *chasing*. ... Take these words and practice them hundreds of times.[2] Be sure that the *ch* is well exploded. The /t/ in front helps to make it so."

[1] Give the patient these words to practice:

shall; shoe; show; shut; ship; shot; shop; shape; shook; shirt; dash; dish; shay; shee; shy; shoe; show; puss-push, push; bus-bush, bush; cass-cash, cash; tuss-tush, tush; dish-shop, shop; dash-shad, shad; push-shall, shall; sash-shape, shape; dish-shed, shed; cash-shell, shell; shut-up; ship-shape; dash-up; dish-it-up.

[2] *chay; chee; chy; choe; chew; chick; chalk; check; cheek; chose; choose; chase; chasing; change; chop; chopping; teach; preacher; search; catch; match; each; choice; chuck; patch; pitch; wretch; reach; chuck-it; chew-it-up; chop-it; short-changed; chop-it-up; hitch-the-catch; check-it-up.*

Unit 12. Aiding Air Intake Through Injection or Tongue Pump (Glossal Press and Glossopharyngeal Press)

"We have worked on /p/, /t/, /k/, /s/, /ʃ/ and /tʃ/, all of which contribute to sending air into the esophagus. The next step is to use the tongue to inject air directly and deliberately into the esophagus. We sometimes call it the pumping method because we move the tongue up sharply to force air out of the mouth and pharynx into the esophagus. (We inject the air without the aid of plosive consonants.) One way of doing this is to start with the tip of the tongue behind the upper front teeth, as in the position /t/; then lift the back of the tongue or rock it backward sharply.[1] When you feel the air entering your esophagus, say *ah*. Watch me do it. Watch my tongue hit the hard palate, then I drop the tongue and bring the air back for an *ah*. You try it; tip of tongue for /t/, push the tongue upward quickly, feel the air going down, then say *ah*. ... Good try, but don't struggle; don't work hard on it.[2] Keep the neck and shoulders relaxed. It's done with the tongue, which pushes the air out of the mouth and pharynx. If you think of opening your throat to receive the air, that will help. Try it again. Rock your tongue back and against the hard palate and say *ah*. ... You are getting good action. Perhaps you should know that some people think they are swallowing air.[3] It's really not a swallow. If there is any resemblance it is just the first part of the swallow. Let's experiment here. Swallow some air and feel what happens to your tongue. ... Did you feel it hit the top of the mouth? ... Now that you felt it, inject the air something like that and say *ah*. ... There you got a better action; I heard air go down and some come up. Here is another tip; close your lips and compress them at the same time as you move your tongue up. ... Still better. You are learning nicely. Now, this time, try the injection and quickly say *ah*. Don't wait; it's like getting the air into a balloon and at once letting it out. You compress it downward and expel it all in one action. So inject and say *ah*. ... Again. ... Again. ... That's good; you got it right that time.

"Place your tongue for /t/, inject and say *tah*.[4]... That's it. Do it again quickly just as you did it. ... Once more, say *tah*. ... Again. ... You are pumping or injecting well because you said a very good vowel in *tah*. You are able to move air by means of plosive sounds and by pumping with the tongue.[5] We will give you another boost of air pressure by using the /s/ and /t/

[1] Draw a picture of the action or refer back to Figure 12, or show the glossal and glossopharyngeal press in Diedrich and Youngstrom.

[2] Emphasize the importance of being at ease in developing injection; the patient must understand that the action is done by the tongue, not the neck muscles.

[3] We prefer not to use the word *swallow*, but it is helpful to some patients. We find it helpful to keep the mouth open wide so that the patient can see the tongue moving up sharply and dropping to a flat position for the production of *ah*. This is for demonstration only. Ordinarily it is better to keep the lips closed to perform a complete injection.

[4] The preplosion pressure for /t/ may be used for the production of /t/ and the tongue pump will produce pressure for the vowel.

[5] This instruction may have to be repeated numerous times before the patient gets it. You may have success only by proceeding through the units immediately following.

combination. Say *stop.*[6] ... *stay.* ... *stoke.* ... *steak.* ... You are getting the vowels much more clearly. Is it easier to inject air now?. ... Say *scat.* ... Good! Say *spot.* ... Walk around the room until the sounds are easy to make. Then work on the vowels with /sp/; say *spay.* ... You first inject, then start /sp/ followed by the vowel.[7] The injection is for the vowel; you compress to make the /sp/ plosives. For words with /st/, you inject, then explode with /st/ and follow with the vowel, like *stick.* Say *stick.* ... Do the same with *skate.* ... Start /sk/, after you inject, and follow with the vowel. Always remember that the work is done inside the mouth, not in the neck. You don't have to raise your eyebrows to inject! You do it most easily when you think of the word and not how much trouble you are going to have. I would like to suggest that you review all of the words we have given you and see how much more effective you are with the aid of the full injection. Let's say the words *state-spate.* ... You need not make a loud klunking sound when you move the air down. If you open your throat and let the air drop down into the esophagus, the klunk will not be heard. Work on making the injection easier and easier. When you learn to do it without thinking, the klunk will be gone. That's your goal. Practice an easy injection at all times."

[6] McClear (1969) uses the *t-ssss-t* method to initiate injection, followed by words that begin with /st/, /sk/, /sp/ etc. This technique is most effective.

[7] See pages 96 and 97 of Diedrich and Youngstrom for the sequential action of injection, plosive sounds and production of vowel. The plosives produce their own compression, but the injection is necessary for the vowel.

Unit 13. Using Minimal Swallow to Demonstrate Injection[1]

"We want to be sure that you get a satisfactory injection, so we are going to violate one of our rules, and that is to show you how to swallow air. Ordinarily we don't do this because some patients use the true swallow and they cannot be good talkers. However, we will have you do a very simple swallow. Will you take a tiny sip of water and hold it in your mouth until I give the signal? ... You use the water to start the swallow but you will swallow

[1] Many contemporary speech clinicians are finally resorting to the use of the genuine swallow action when the patient is unable to inject in the ways presented thus far. The possibility of this action being retained need not disturb anyone, because the demand for rapid speech production prevents retention of this habit.

a lot of air with it, which can be used to say *ah*. Get ready, swallow the water and immediately say *ah*. ... You swallowed but didn't get the air back up.[2] That's of great importance, otherwise you don't talk. It's done in one action, taking in air and bringing it back up as you speak.[3] Really, you reverse the column of air, first going down, then coming back and up. Take another sip. Now swallow and say *ah*. ... Let's do it this way. Put your hand on me right under my rib cage. That shows when my diaphragm moves down, and then the muscles tighten up to move the air out of the stoma. When you swallow the water and air, tighten your abdominal muscles a bit, and that will help the air come back up. Once more, take a sip, swallow, tighten the abdomen and say *ah*. ... That was it! Now quickly say *ah* again. ... Again. ... Let's do the swallow without the sip just like you did with these last sounds but do it fast; in fast and out fast is our goal. So say *ah* very fast. ... Now say *pah* very fast. ... Now *stop*. ... That shows your greatest progress. The next step is to make sure that you do this faster speed with every word you say. So let's practice saying the word just as quickly as you can when I give it to you. In fast and out fast is what we want,[4] but don't tighten up; it's all done in the mouth with the tongue. Say *ah*. ... *pah*. ... *tah*. ... *kah*. ... *pop*. ... *top* ... Now try two sounds together. Say *pop-top* quickly. ... That's good. Say *stop* five times, injecting for each one. ... Now you are getting faster action. If you remember that the tongue works faster than you realize, you can get the sound down and back in less than a second. Now, you can review all of the words again and notice how much easier it is to say them."

To the speech clinician: If the patient has learned by plosive-injection techniques up to this point, he need not be trained in the inhalation method that is to be given next. However, since some

[2] If the water comes back out of the patient's nose, it indicates that his soft palate is not closing for injection.

[3] If the patient doesn't say *ah* but a moment later belches, say, "That's something like what we want, but you use it to say the word." Then have him repeat the act.

[4] For information on the injection technique, consult Diedrich and Youngstrom; M.C.L. Greene; Snidecor 1968; and the manuals listed in the Appendix.

patients use both injection and inhalation, it is worthwhile to demonstrate the method. You may find that the patient is good at this technique, merely from having worked with the previous techniques. Furthermore, he may wish to add to his skills.

Unit 14. Air Intake: Inhalation

To the speech clinician: This unit is intended for the patient who has been unable to establish esophageal voice up to this point. After he has learned to inhale, return to Unit 7 and proceed to Unit 11.

"Here is another method of moving air into the esophagus.[1] Can you yawn? Some people do it easily. Try it. ... Don't work hard on it. A yawn means you are relaxing, letting yourself go. Do it this way: Put the tip of the tongue behind the lower teeth. Open your mouth widely and smile broadly, as if you are enjoying it.[2] Drop the back of the tongue as you breathe in air, keeping the tip against the teeth. Feel the cool air move into your throat as you breathe through your stoma. It may feel as if you are sucking air in your throat as well as your stoma, as a smoker can do. So open your mouth from front to back to draw all the air in that you can. Think of opening up the throat as you yawn. ... Do it a little faster as you yawn, and say *ah*. ... Do it a little faster and say *ah* as soon as you feel the air has entered the throat. ...

"Let's do something positive that will help you take in air. Stick out your chin, or jerk your head backward as you inhale.[3] It will help to open the esophagus. Watch me. ... Now do it. ... You heard and felt the air go down, didn't you? ... Fine. Now, breathe in fast as you jerk your head. ... Good. That was a good sound that came back up.

"Here is another definite help to get air

[1] Consult Diedrich and Youngstrom; M.C.L. Greene; Hodson and Oswald; and Snidecor 1968 for different methods of developing air intake by inhalation.

[2] Proof of success is when you really yawn!

[3] Moore (1957) suggested that jerking the head back opens the esophagus. This has been an effective method. After the technique has been fixed, the patient should be taught to reduce the head-jerk movement. Some patients discover that they do better on inhalation if they turn the head to one side as they jerk backward. Each patient finds for himself the most effective action.

down. As you inhale, sniff air through your nose.[4] Some people do this quite well. They can sniff to smell roses; it brings back their sense of smell for a moment. So, do this: close the lips and sniff sharply through your nose.[5] ... Good, but you lifted your shoulders and bulged your neck muscles. Once more. ... We'll have to change your breathing method. You are lifting your shoulders and your chest. That means you produce tension in the neck muscles which help do the lifting. You can't inject easily or inhale that way. Do it this way: Put your hand on me just below my rib cage; I call it the triangle.[6] As I inhale, you will feel my abdomen (the triangle) and your hand moving outward. That means the diaphragm is being pulled downward to allow air to enter the lungs. When I breathe out, your hand moves back as my abdomen moves in.[7]

"Put your hand on your own epigastric area, as you did on mine. Breathe in; see it and feel the abdomen move out. Now sigh and notice that it moves back in. ... Let's inhale this new way, as you open up your throat and sniff through the nose. It will help air enter the esophagus. Inhale fast and then say *ah*. ... Let's record what you can say. Say *ah*. ... Sniff and say *ah-ah*. ... Now sniff and say *pat*. ... *skip*. ... *spot*. ... OK. ... *Inhale* and say *pah-tah*. ... *Inhale and say pah-tah-kah*. ... Say *tisket-tasket*. Let's play it back. ... Did you notice that the sniff gave you more volume? ... That was because it helped you get more air into the esophagus. From now on, make it routine to sniff air through your nose before you say a word. You may also get some air through your mouth if you keep the lips parted slightly.[8] If a person greets you, sniff lightly and inject, then return the greeting. If anyone asks you a question, sniff before you say a word. You will always get more air that way. And avoid the habit of lifting your shoulders or tightening

[4] Read how Diedrich and Youngstrom handle the sniff (page 112 of their book).

[5] If the patient has been brought through the entire series up to this point, and has done well, and has no need of inhaling for air intake, practice with him on the sniff technique and henceforth always remind him to take in air with a sniff (prior to or with injection, or with the inhalation method) if he is to use it.

[6] The epigastric area or the substernal area.

[7] See also Unit 5 on relaxation and breathing.

[8] Of course, the patient is getting lung air through the stoma.

the neck muscles. They don't help; rather they hinder good voice."

Unit 15. Aiding Expulsion by Expiration

"We've talked a lot about how to get air in but have said little about how to get it out in order to help your speech. Put your hand on me again right under my rib cage. I will breathe in and then I will push your hand and mine against my abdomen. ... You heard me say *ah* as I contracted my abdomen, that is, it moved inward. We don't push our abdomen in hard every time we speak out. Rather, the muscles naturally contract and put the abdomen under tension. At the same time the action pushes the diaphragm upward. That is the action that contributes to the outward flow of air. So every time we take in air we must firm the abdomen to move the air out. That gives you fluency and audibility of voice."

To the speech clinician: At this point, give Periodic Test 2 (page 97).

Phase III. Developing Voiced Sounds

Unit 16. Sustaining Air for Two Syllables

"You can get a lot of compression by saying /p/, /t/ and /k/ in succession.[1] Feel the air pressure in your throat and explode each consonant in succession. ... Don't use voice; don't strain your face muscles on the /k/.[2] Don't squint your eyes just because you are trying to sustain the voice for several sounds. Once more: say the unvoiced /p/, /t/, /k/. ... Good. Now, say /p/, /t/, /k/. ... Good. Now, say /p/, /t/, /k/, *ah.* ... Again. ... Better. Now say *pah-tah-kah,*[3] all with one air-charge. ... You must say these three syllables hundreds of times. Every fifteen minutes, say some. When you are out walking, say them; while you are putting on your shirt, say them. It is fast tongue action with a good explosion that counts. It

[1] Whispering is not allowed by some clinicians. This is really not whispering; it is like an unvoiced *puh-puh-puh.* Each consonant helps to move air backward.

[2] Strive for perfection of the explosion first; however, the tongue can manipulate the sounds rapidly without loss of compression, after much practice.

[3] The dash between words in a series indicates that the entire series is produced with one air-charge and without pause.

will give you confidence that you are winning.

"Now that you are getting a good *pah-tah-kah*, try your skill on two words. Try these: *pat-pit. ... pie-pay. ... pet-put. ... pot-pie. ... tay-tea. ... tie-toe. ... pup-pipe. ... pick-it-up. ... pick-pocket .... tic-tac-toe. ... pocketbook. ... pep-it-up.* ... Practice this list of words.[4] Try to talk with your family, using at least two syllables at a time. Speak a sentence with not more than two words or syllables with one air-charge. Do this and you will soon discard all writing."

[4] Words for practice:

tay-tea; tie-toe; pot-pie; pick-pack; teacup; catspaw; top-cot; pick-tick; tack-it; tic-tac; tic-tac-toe; pick-it; pick-it-up; pocket; pickpocket; pocket-book; pep-it-up; tip-it-up; shake-it; dish-it; dish-it-up; keep-it; keep-it-up; chuck-it; chock-it; stop-it; stop-it-up; shake-it-up; shake-it-out; keep-at-it.

Unit 17. Prolonging the Vowel Tone

To the speech clinician: Now that the patient has acquired skill at injection and/or inhaling for air intake, aided especially by the different plosive consonants, we will concentrate on developing his ability to communicate. Our immediate goal, therefore, is to establish skill in producing the vowels and then the voiced consonants.[1]

"Before we get started on the next lesson, let's find out what words you can be using at home.[2] Will you please say *no?* ... And try to say *yes.* ... Say *How are you?* ... Do you know why you are having trouble saying them?. ... Because they don't have any plosive sounds to help you say them. Voiced sounds have to be initiated by injecting air, so we are going to work on vowels, which are the voiced sounds; also, some unvoiced consonants have voiced partners. Let's have the name of your son. ... Patrick? Good. But you call him Pat? ... That's a good plosive sound. So say it. ... Good. What is your wife's name? ... Katherine. Do you call her Kate? ... Then say *Kate.* ... From now on use their names frequently to get experience. What do you call your dog? ... Chip? Fine! Another plosive. Practice calling him when you want to take him out. Bring the

[1] From now on, the patient will be exposed to a large vocabulary of words. He should be urged to practice them hundreds of times. If you find a need for more words consult the manuals listed in the Appendix.

[2] With every lesson from now on inquire about the patient's progress in talking. Have him bring phrases and sentences that are commonly used in the home and at work. Go over these in order to help him practice with words that will increase his working vocabulary.

names of your friends, and a list of words you want to use around home.

"We are going to use the plosive sounds to help you prolong some of the vowels.[3] Will you start *pah* and hold the vowel several seconds? Do it like this: *paaaaaaaaaaaaaa.* ... You faded out quickly but held on to it long enough to show you are making progress. Try it once more, but don't fight it; stop before you exhaust all of your air; otherwise you tighten up. Once more, *paaaaaaa.* ... That's better but don't squeeze the sound as the air fades; just stop. Don't strain with your neck muscles. Just stop trying when the air fades.[4] All of the action is done within the mouth; the tongue compresses and injects the air, then it articulates the speech sounds. Once more; sniff and hold the vowel in *paaaaaaaa.* That was better right to the last sound. Do the same with /t/: *taaaaaaaa.* ... Good.[5] Let's try *kaaaaaaaaaaa.* ... You don't need to make a face and frown when you speak. Be at ease and let the tongue inject and then bring the sound out. Once more: *kaaaaaaaaa.* Let's try sah: *saaaaaaaaaa.* ... That was quite strong. How about *chah?* ... Another good one. Try *shah;* hold it two seconds if you can. ... Pretty close! Let's try some other vowels. Prolong each vowel ending as long as you can. *Pay.* ... *pea.* ... *pie.* ... *poe.* ... *poo.* ... Prolong the same vowels with /t/. ... You are getting stronger vowels. Do the same with /k/. ... Fine."

[3] It's wise not to say "as long as you can," because the patient may get the idea that he has to strain to talk.

[4] You may have to repeat the technique with the same sound several times before moving on to another. This is a critical point in developing vowels. It may be necessary to go back to tongue injection exercises. Our experience is that at this point, the patient may already have used injection to produce vowels. The best technique for producing the initial vowel, which is difficult, is to glide from a final vowel to the initial vowel. If a patient has difficulty with a vowel, suggest that he say it with a plosive and then carry the image of the vowel to the initial position in a spontaneous manner.

[5] Other exercises:

pa-taaaaa; pa-kaaaa;
ta-paaaa; ta-kaaaaa;
ka-paaaa; taaa-ka; saaaaa-ta;
kaaaaa-sa; chaaaa-shaaa;
soo-sooooo; see-seeeeee; sigh-
siiiiiii; say-saaaaaaaa;
shoo-chooooo;
shay-shaaaaaaa;
stayayayayay;
skee-skeeeeeee; spee-speeeee,
spy-spyyyyyyyy;
stee-steeeee; stoe-stooooooo.

Unit 18. Developing the Initial Vowel

"You have already spoken many vowels with the plosive words. Now, we will show you how you can do them without a plosive sound and in the initial position. This means that there is no plosive to help you. You have to make a full injection of air before you can make the sound. You can do it more easily by getting the feeling for producing the sound in the final position and immediately saying it again as an initial vowel. But you must inject before you say it the second time. Try this: *pea-ee.* ... Again. ... *pea-ee, ee.* ... The last one should have had an injection before you produced it. Try it once more: *pea-ee, ee.* ... Good. Put a /t/ to the *vowel so we say pea-ee, eat.* ... Good. Next we will say *pea-eat, eat.* ... Fine. Say *eat.* ... Again. You have the initial vowel. Let's try some other vowels: *page-age, age.* ... *pout-out, out.* ... *cup-up, up.* ... *pant-ant, ant.* ... Whenever you start a word with a vowel, you must inject. When you start with a plosive consonant, you may get some air in with the plosive action, but it is better to inject before you start the word and take advantage of both the plosive and the initial injection.

"Let's practice with the vowels in the initial and final positions. Say *ahtah.* ... The same vowel with *apa.* ... *ahkah.* ... *oepoe.* ... *oopoo.* ... *oesoe.* ... *aychay.* ... *iepie.* ... *ate-eat.* ... *up-ape.* ... *it-at.* ... *eel-heal.* ... *eke-ache.* ... *ash-each.* ... *owl-oil.* ...[1]

"Here's the easy way to say: *How are you?* You say: *'ow ah eeoo?* You don't hear the /h/ anyway, and most persons would not notice that you left out some sounds. Try it. ... You left off the /j/ (*y*) sound in *you.* The sound is made by first saying *ee* and gliding quickly to *oo* as you sharply raise your tongue. Try it: *ee-oo.* ... Now shorten the first vowel, say it quickly and glide to *oo.* That's better. Now say *How are you?* See if it is easier to say, rather, *'Ow ah eeoo?* ... Good. Try some more words with /j/: *yes.* ... Do it this way: *ee-yes, yes.* ... *ee-you.* ... *yacht.* ... *yoke.* ... *ye.* ... *yaw.* ... *yaks.* ... *yeggs.* ... *yeast.* ... *yet.* ...

"While we are working on *yes,* we should work on its opposite, *no.* We'll handle the /n/

[1] If the patient has trouble with an initial vowel, he should first say it with a plosive and then alone. Have the patient practice these words many times with an easy injection, until it is automatic:

pea-ee; pea-ee; eat; page-age, age; pout-out, out; cup-up, up; tout-out, out; pat-at; pop-hop; pitch-itch; pearl-earl; pan-an; sand-and; pit-it; pow-how; tact-act; pate-ate; tape-ape; cap-apt; taught-ought; Pam-am; pock-hock; book-hook; task-ask; Tod-odd; totes-oats, tear-ear; tome-home; putt-hut; peat-heat.

sail-ail; ail, ail, ail, ail, call-all, all, all, all, all; pit-it, it, it, it, it, it; stout-out, out, out, out, out.

eat it up; ate it up; act it out; Are you OK? How do you do? How are you?

ah-tah; ahpah; ahkah; oepoe; oopoo; oesoe; aychay; iepie; ate-eat; up-ape; it-at; out-oil.

up and at 'em; at a boy; up and out; aim at it; pouch; pooch; poach; patch; peach; pitch; pop; poop; pip; pap; peep; pup; head; heed; hood; hod; had; hide; arch; ark; attic; cut; caught; cot; kit; skeet; scat; scoot.

Otto ought to pay up. A tip-top cop caught the ape.

sound later, but for the present regard it as a voiced sound made when you put your tongue up for saying /n/. So say *no. ... not. ... yes and no. ... I say No! ... You say Yes! I say How are are you? ... You say How are you?*

"We've forgotten one of the most important words in your life: *I*. That really is two vowels blended: /aɪ/, like *ah-ee*. Say it. ... Say *ice. ... kite. ... tight. ... bite. ... sight. ... tike. ...* Now say: *I see you. ... I saw you. ... You and I. ... I say No! ...* You may pause and inject if you can't say the entire phrase in one air intake: *Yes, I can cook. ...* Take this list, and say the words hundreds of times.[2] Be accurate!"

Unit 19. Voicing Plosive Sounds

"Please read the lists of words with vowels that you took home. ... You are getting very good prolongation on some of the vowels. Be sure to sniff and inject before each word or pair of words that begins with a vowel. Did you have any trouble with initial vowels? ... Keep up the practice many times a day and you will will be getting greater confidence in talking.

"Now that you have good vowel sounds, which means that you have the ability to produce all voiced sounds, we will work on voiced plosives. Some consonants are simply noises or friction sounds, or explosive sounds, none of which are voiced. But many of them have partners which are voiced, such as /p/ and /b/, /t/ and /d/, /k/ and /g/, and /s/ and /z/. We will do the sound /b/, which is paired with /p/. You produce it by adding voice to the action for /p/.[1] We will start with /b/ at the end of

[2] The patient should say as many words as he can on one air-charge:

I; you; yes; take; cook; Yes, you can; If you can; If he can; can you cook? It's your hat; I can cook, too; Yes, he can; Can you take it? Can your cat eat it? Can't you eat it? Can't you talk? Yes, I can talk. Yes, I took it.

yet; yacht; yoke; ye; yaw; yes; yaks; yeast; yea; yew.

If the patient cannot say two words per air-charge, have him say one word for each injection. He must get a good injection when there is an initial vowel.

Some patients will require considerable repetition and review of preceding exercises. Aim for accuracy; not loudness.

[1] The voiced plosive requires a complex action of intrapharyngeal compression for the plosive phases and tongue pump or injection for the voiced phases. Both aspects must be present when the voiced plosive is in the final position; the tendency is to fail to produce voice, and this leaves only the unvoiced plosive action, or a simple approximation of the articulated position. Hence, much work must be done on final voiced and unvoiced sounds.

a word because it will be associated with a preceding vowel. Say this word pair: *cap-cab.* You must inject before you start the first sound /k/, which may supply a slight amount of additional air to the esophagus. Then you sustain the voiced part for both the *a* and *b.* Say *cap-cab.* ... Listen for the voiced /b/ at the end of the word. You must expel vibrations from the esophagus long enough to make an audible /b/. Try *cap-cab* once more. ... I heard the /b/ much better. Hold this TOK-BAK[2] against your ears. It will help you to hear the /b/ louder. Once more: *cap-cab.* Some people just put the lips together but don't explode. The sound must be exploded. Say *cup-cub.* ... *sop-sob.* ... *cop-cob.* ... *dap-dab, dab.* ... *mop-mob, mob.* ... *age-Abe, Abe.* ... *coop-cube, cube.* ... Let's try some words with /b/ in the initial position. Say *pah-bah.* ... *pea-bee.* ... *pat-bat.* ... *pit-bit.* ... *putt-but, but.* ... *peet-beet, beet.* ... *peep-beet, beet.* ... *pab-bab, bab.* ... *pub-bub, bub.* ... Try initial vowels with /b/: *ape-Abe.* ... *eep-eeb.* ... *ie-ieb.* ... *oep-oeb.* ... *oop-oob.* ... Then say the vowels after the /b/: *bay-bee.* ... *bye-boo.* ... *boe.* ... *cop-bob, bob.* ... *cub-bub, bub.* ... *sub-bus, bus.* ... *tab, bab, bab.* ... Take these words lists and do the words hundreds of times. Make up sentences with them.[3]

✗ *To the speech clinician:* At this point, give Periodic Test 3 (page 97).

"The sound /d/ is paired with the plosive consonant /t/. Let's do these pairs: *pat-pad.* ... *at-add.* ... *ate-aid.* ... *state-staid.* ... *tied-died.* ... *spite-spied.* ... *hat-had.* ... Let's try some initial sounds of /d/. *to-do, do.* ... *Ted-dead, dead.* ... *taupe-dope, dope.* ... *tick-Dick, Dick.* ... *tip-dip, dip.* ... *tyke-dike, dike.* ... *day-dee-die.* ... *doe-do-dow.* ... Try some phrases: *Ted did it.* ... *Tad did it.* ... *Dick caught it.* ... *Dad tied up the cow.* ..."[4]

[2] See the Appendix.

[3] *cap-cab; cup-pub; sop-sob; cop-cob; dap-dab; mop-mob; bop-bob; bay; bee; bye; boe; boo; pat-bat; pit-bit; putt-but; peet-beet; peep-beep; pus-bus; pub-bub; bite; bought; butt it; bag; back; bed; big; boat; bug; bus; boy; by; be; bat; baby; bye-bye; Bud bought it; Bob bit it; Buck took the bus.*

cob-bob, bob; cub-bub, bub; tub-bab, bab; sub-bus, bus; sob-boss, boss; dab-bab, bab; cap, cab, bab.

Buy it up; batter up; Better take a cab; Bub bought two cubs; Buck up, Bob; Bet a buck; Two boats on the bay.

[4] Have the patient take these home for practice:

pat-pad; at-add; ate-aid; state-staid; tied-died; spite-spied; hat-had; too-do-do; Ted-dead, dead; taupe-dope, dope; tick-Dick, Dick; tip, dip, day; dee; doe; doo; tyke-dike; tout-doubt; tuck-duck, duck; toes-does, does; too-do, do; did; dud; dice; dies; dip; dot; desk; dusk; dock; sad; said; stayed; bad; bed; Bud; code; toad; goad; good; could; cued; sobbed; bobbed; bedded; busted;; dusted; Dad did it; Ted did it, too; Put Ted's bed out; Dick caught Ted in bed; I had to do it.

Unit 20. Pairing Plosive /k/ with voiced /g/

"The voiced plosive consonant /g/ is paired with voiceless /k/. Since /g/ is voiced, be sure to make it audible by saving the air supply and slightly exaggerating it at first. Try this pair: *back-bag.* ... Get the voiced sound. Hear it; *feel it.* Once more, *back-bag.* ... *beck-beg.* ... *dock-dog.* ... Make a definite contrast of the /k/ with the voiced /g/. *Dick-dig, dig.* ... *pick-pig, pig.* ... *sack-sag, sag.* ... *puck-pug, pug.* ... Now we'll carry over from the final /g/ in the first word to the initial /g/ in the second word, then clinch the kinesthetic image for initial /g/ by repeating the second word. You may hesitate and inject before you say the final word. Try this trio: *tag-gate, gate.* ... *pig-gape, gape.* ... *pug-guppy, guppy.* ... *lag-gag, gag.* ... *cog-got, got.* ... *keg-get, get.* ... *get-going.* ... *Kate got it.* ... *Dick bagged a tiger.* ... *A big game of puck.* ... *I gave it to Doc's goat.* ... *The cutter sagged at the dock.* ... *Tad dug it up.* ... *Pug tugged at it.* ... *Pegleg got a wooden leg.* ... *biggest egg.* ... *Go east; go west; go where it's best.* ... *Take this list home.*"[1]

To the speech clinician: Discuss with the patient the possibility of discarding his pad and pencil and participating in family conversation.

[1] Give these words to the patient. You furnish others according to his needs:

back-bag, bag; beck-beg, beg; dock-dog, dog; dick-dig, dig; peck-peg, peg; sack-sag, sag; puck-pug, pug; big-pig, pig; tuck-tug, tug; rock-rag, rag; tack-tag, tag; buck-bug, bug; kick-gig, gig; tag-gate, gate; pig-gape, gape; pug-guppy, guppy; lag-gag, gag; cog-got, got; keg-get, get.

go; goat; got; get; gate; gay; good; goose; geese; guess; beg; peg; big; biggest; egg; leg; dig; pig; pug; hoggy; boggy; buggy.

The patient should inhale before each of the following words or phrases:

dig it; guess what; Tad dug it up; biggest hog; deepest bog; Pug tugged at it; Go get big pig; Pegleg got a wooden leg; Get going; Get it; I gave it to Dick's goat; The cutter sagged at the dock.

Unit 21. Producing Voiced Pairs of /s/, /ʃ/ and /tʃ/

"The consonants /s/ and /z/ are also paired. First sustain /s/ at the end of a word and then add voice. This is done by injecting for the voiced part of the sound. Thus, *passssssz.* ...[1] Try it once more. You might get enough air from the esophagus from the supply injected by /s/, but let's assume that there is not enough air. For practice only we charge air to produce the /z/. Do it this way: *passsss,* inject and say /z/. This time, sniff sharply as soon as you terminate the /s/: *passsss,* sniff, inject, say /z/. ...

[1] Since final /z/ follows a vowel, the patient should endeavor to sustain enough air from the preceding injection to voice the /z/. But in order to train the patient, we emphasize /z/ by having him inject for it.

That's good. Try some other words. Say *hiss-his*. ... You must prolong the phonation of the vowel to produce the voice of the /z/. Once more: *hiss-his*. ... Get a good voiced /z/. Say *his*. ... *peace-peas, peas*. ... *face-faze, faze*. ... *noose-news, news*. ... *dice-dies, dies*. ... *this-these, these*. ... *pecks-pegs, pegs*. ... *picks-pigs, pigs*. ... *his-zig, zig*. ... *his-zag, zag*. ... *zig-zag*. ... *his-zip, zip*. ... *his-zap, zap*. ... *zip-zap*. ... *Jack tugs at his dogs*. ... Good work. Take this list home to work on.[2]

"Have you been counting? By this time, you ought to be counting every day up to 100. And the same with the ABC's. Do as many as you can with one air-charge. You have your work cut out for you.

"The voiced partner for /ʃ/ (*sh*) is /ʒ/ (zh), as in *measure*. Start with the word mash and then say *measure; mash, measure*. ... Try it this way: *mash-maize, measure*. ... *lash-laize, leisure*. ... Try it this way: *mash-masher, measure*. ... Good. Try *lash-lasher, leisure*. ... That is better. Say *visit-vision*. ... *fission-vision*. ... *adhesive-adhesion*. ... *usual-usury*. ... Practice the words on this list carefully.[3]

"The voiced partner of /tʃ/ (*ch*) is /dʒ/ (*dj*), as in *judge*. This means that you use /d/ instead of /t/ to blend. Say *batch-badge*. ... *rich-ridge*. ... *etch-edge*. ... *age-jade-jade*. ... *age-jade, jade*. ... *edge-judge, judge*. ... *urge-jerk, jerk*. ... *edge-jet, jet*. ... *January*. ... *June*. ... *July*. ... *John and Jim*. ... *Judge George J. January*. ... *page-age*. ... *cage-wage*. ... *page-gage* ... *huge-budget*. ... *sage-judge*. ... *hodge-podge*. ... *Watch out for the ridge on the bridge*. ... *The judge completed his decision*. ... *Enjoy a joyous July*. ... You have no trouble with these. Work on this list many times."[4]

[2] *zoo; zest; fuss-fuzz; say-zay; see-zee; sigh-sighs; sighs-size; zip-zap-zup; dogs-bogs, bogs; hiss-his, his; peace-peas, peas; face-faze, faze; noose-news, news; dice-dies, dies; this-these, these; pecks-pegs, pegs; picks-pigs, pigs.*

Jack tugs with his dogs; "Pros" at the zoo don't tease the zebras; What does Charles desire for the holidays?

sues-zoos, zoos; says-zest, zest; nose-zone, zone; sing-zing, zing, zing; pigs-zig-zag; heroes-zeroes, zeroes.

[3] *masher-measure, measure; use-you-usual, usual; lasher-leisure; decisive-decision; fish-vision; adhesive-adhesion; visual; vision; usual; seizure; azure; evasion; derision; rouge; prestige; garage; corsage; loge; camouflage.*

[4] *jay; jee; jie; joe; Jew; jog; joke; jar; badge; ridge; edge; bridge; judge; George; jug; James; John; Jim; Jack; January; June; July; enjoy; object; page; jig; agitate; cage; wage; ledge; page; gage; huge; budge; sage; hodge-podge.*

It is good to jest, to turn a joke, but not to make a trade of jesting; Jim has jam on his jacket; Watch out for the ridge on the bridge; The judge completed his decision; Jack shot a badger under the bridge.

Keep helping the patient to build up his vocabulary. If he intends to return to his job, have him list words commonly used on the job. Make up sentences with them.

Unit 22. Semi-Vowels: /l/, /r/, /m/, /n/ and /ŋ/ (ng)

"We don't have pairs for /l/ and /r/. They are voiced as are vowels. You have advanced to the point where you do not need detailed explanations of speech sounds. However, there is a need for articulating these well. Let's run right through some /l/ words. Say *lay-lee. ... lie-low. ... loo-let. ... lad-late-like. ... lock-collar. color-dollar. ... yellow-pillow. .. foolish-fellow. ... blow-blue. ... alley. ... hold-told. ... yellow-pallor. ... luscious-lily. ... Pull up close to the mall. ... He filled the leaky jugs with oil. ... He was black and blue from the blows. ... pleasant-place. ... Let the air blow out of the tires. ...* Do the word lists many times.[1]

"The sound /r/ is made by curling up the tongue slightly so that the air flows over its point. Say *ran-ragged. ... really-rich. ... roaming-roads. ... large-hammer. ... chair-ripe-stripe. ... tare-tear. ... rare-rear. ... roaring-rally. ... ripe-fruit. ... terrible-reaper. ... cracked-mirror. ...* Read the words on the list.[2]

"The nasal sounds /m/, /n/ and /ŋ/ are made with the soft palate closed in order to maintain compression. Nevertheless, the sounds must be pronounced as usual, lips closed for /m/ and open for /n/ and /ŋ/. So let's say *mamma-papa. ... many-times. ... much-more. ... moon-drum-plum. ... moon-maid. ... home-made. ... lemonade. ... Christmas-time. ... Are you coming home tomorrow? ... almost every time. ... pommel of the saddle. ... blossom-time. ... farmer in the meadow. ... Mamma made some jam for company. ... capitol-dome. Let's go to our summer home. ... The hummingbird hummed near the barn. ... Now is the time for all good men to come to the aid of the party. ... in-and-out. ... into-onto. ... night and day. ... downtown at noon. ... again and again. ... dinner-time. ... Can you can them in the new aluminum cans? ... nook and cranny. ... nice and never noisy. ...* Work on the list for practice.[3]

[1] Word lists for /l/:

lay; lad; late; like; lake; lie; lock; color; collar; dollar; fellow; pillow; yellow; pallor; light; loom; locust; luscious; list; likely; gull; swell; pill; pull; pall; alley; pulse; silly.

lay-lee-lie; low-loo; lad-late-like; lock-collar; yellow-pallor; luscious-lily; foolish-fellow; Pull-up-close to the mall; He filled the leaky jugs with oil; He was black and blue from the blows; It was a pleasant place; Let the air blow out of the tires.

[2] *ran; rag; rap; ready; rich; cheer; chair; ripe; road; rope; lay; lad; late; like; lake; lie; lock; color; collar; dollar; roar; arrow; sparrow; rural; mural; already; sorrel; relish; rate; relapse; red; raze; rush; richer; racketeer; railroad; recorder; roaring-rally; ripe-fruit; rolling-roads; raring-roadster; rooster-breader; rare-dealer; Jack the Ripper; Put rip-rap along the river; Robbers ran rapidly to the railroad yard.*

[3] *mamma; summer; hammer; almost; moon; much; drum; plum; home; tame; name; came; lame; tram; clam; climb; am; beaming; timber; pommel; lemon; company; empty; sometime; animal; Christmas; some; same; soon; come; summer; home; Mamma made me some jam; The humming bird hummed near the barn; Now is the time for all good men to come to the aid of the party; Mamma moved to the summer home; spasm; prism; blossom.*

"The /ŋ/ sound is difficult to make. You must make a positive action with the back of the tongue to make it intelligible. Try this: *sing-song. ... sung-rung-rang. ... ping-pong-king. ... wing-ring-bang. ... longing and ringing ... sitting and thinking. ... knitting and blinking. ... clinging and sinking. ... coming and going. ... Sally sang for the King in the gallery. ... singing of angels with wings. ... seizing and teasing and ringing. ... running, walking and jumping.* ... Read the list for practice many times."[4]

[4] *nice; noose; news; name; noon; known; noun; town; down; round; pin; tone; tine; pain; den; dent; dint; pan; pants; nun; need; nod; funny brown man; singing a song; night and noon; green and sand background; many new plants in the spring garden; Don't fence me in; Anne may spend the night with a new friend; Chickens stand in the barn on rainy days; sitting and thinking; coming and going; knitting and blinking; clinging and singing; tossing and ringing; singing of angels in the wings; running and walking and jumping.*

Unit 23. Remaining Consonants: /f/, /v/, /θ/ (*th*), /ð/ (*th*), /w/ and /hw/

"The sound /f/ is paired with its voiced sound /v/. Say these words: *fat-vat. ... life-live. ... gift-give. ... sift-sieve. ... safe-save. ... staff-stave. ... strife-strive. ... few-view. ... cuffer-cover. ... fine-vine. ... valley-view ... fine-value. ... heifer-heaver. ... leaf-lever. ... Did you ever live in Valley View?* ... Make up some sentences with words that have /f/ and /v/. Read these words.[1]

"The *th* sound is paired; /θ/ is voiceless and /ð/ is voiced. Try these: *thin-then. ... thought-though. ... cloth-clothe. ... bath-bathe. ... breath-breathe. ... father-mother. ... grandmother-grandfather. ... Leather boots are fine in wet*

[1] *fat; fit; feet; food; ford; fight; fetch; off; if; leaf; life; knife; puff; laugh; cough; careful; coffee; office; safely; safety; staff; view; visit; vine; violet; valley; value; vegetable; vote; vow; ever; over; never; clever; clover; river; favor; favorite; evening; heavy; gave; cave; have; heave; hove; rover; fine-vine; very-few; valley-view; fine-value; over and over; few views; Save and be safe; Did you ever live in Valley View?*

weather. ... It's smooth as a feather. ... Practice the words on the list.[2]

"The sounds /w/ and /hw/ will sound alike because the speaker does not have lung air to furnish the fast air movement for the /h/ aspect of /hw/. Whatever air is available comes from the intraoral-pharyngeal cavities and is not related to the expelled air after injection. If you can get a movement of the tongue and lips as for a whistle, you can develop the sound. So it is important for you to try to whistle, as some speakers do. Can you? ... Practice on it as often as you think about it. Blow tissue paper and feathers off a flat surface. Let's practice some contrasting words: Say *watt-what. ... Wye-why. ... we-whee. ... woe-whoa. ... wit-whit. ... wide-white ... wen-when. ... weal-wheel. ... wet-whet. ... wile-while. ... witch-which. ... heat-wheat. ... hare-where. ... ham-wham. ... height-white. ... wail-whale. ... hail-whale. ... The wheel whirled off the shaft. ... What whim made him take a swim? ... Whither and whether thou goes. ...* Practice on these words and be sure to hear the difference between the /w/ and the /hw/ sounds."[3]

[2] *thin; think; thank; thing; three; thirty; teeth; cloth; tooth; faith; birth; north; month; fifty-fourth; faith; nothing; thirst; this; they; them; that; though; the; those; than; then; therewith; oath; gather; clothe; soothe; within; either; nothing; anything; youth; both; path; mouth; teeth; tooth; thought-though; cloth-clothe; bath-bathe; breath-breathe; father; mother; grandmother-grandfather; father-mother; Leather boots are fine in wet weather; It's smooth as a feather.*

[3] *oh-whoa; air-where; am-wham; is-whiz; aisle-while; ease-wheeze; wit-whit; itch-which; wail-whale; wile-while; hot-what; his-whiz; Wye-why; watt-what; we-whee; wide-white; wet-whet; The wheel whirled off the shaft; What whim made him take a swim? Whither thou goest I will go.*

To the speech clinician: At this point, give Periodic Test 4 (page 98).

Phase IV. Developing Fluency

Unit 24. Fluency Through Longer Words

To the speech clinician: In order to keep "the utterance flowing" (Van Riper) and to keep the "uninterrupted, effortless esophageal speech" (Berlin 1965a) that is present in the fluency of good esophageal speakers, we present the patient with longer and longer words and phrases. By adding more and more syllables to a word, we stimulate the patient to increase the number of syllables he can produce on one air intake. Under no circumstances should the patient get the impression that he should rush. Let his tongue and breathing do the work. Instruct the patient to sniff and/or inject before each group of syllables presented—for example, before *like,* before *likely* and before *likelihood.*

like	likely	likelihood	
in	invade	invasion	
prop	proper	property	
part	partner	partnership	
ex	extra	extricate	extricated
pre	prefer	preference	preferential
in	intim	intimate	intimation
all	allure	alluring	alluringly
spec	specu	speculate	speculation
re	relay	relation	relationship
merch	merchant	merchandise	merchandising
des	desper	desperate	desperado
miss	missile	misalign	misalignment
in	innu	innuen	innuendo
ale	alien	alienate	alienation
insig	insignif	insignifi	insignificance
precip	precipi	precipitous	precipitousness
aman	amanu	amanuen	amanuensis
delib	deliber	deliberate	deliberation
civil	civilize	civiliza	civilization
predom	predomin	predominate	predomination
advis	advisa	advisable	advisability
veterin	veterinar	veterinary	veterinarian
transfer	transfera	transferable	transferability
particu	particular	particularize	particularization
respons	responsi	responsible	responsibility
preternat	preternatur	preternatural	preternaturalize
para	parallel	parallelo	parallelogram
appre	apprehen	apprehensi	apprehensibility
appre	appreci	appreciate	appreciative

Unit 25. Increasing the Fluency of Nonplosive-Laden Words

To the speech clinician: Words that are plosive-laden are easier to say than words that have no plosive sounds. We wish to demonstrate to the patient the difference between such words by requesting him to say a word that has a plosive sound followed by a word that has no plosive sounds. In our clinical experience, speakers appear to be able to say the nonplosive-laden word more easily after experiencing fluency in the preceding plosive-laden word. They apparently make the effort to maintain a forward flow of sound, in spite of the injections they have to make. This experience applies to patients who inject; we have had no experience in this respect from inhalers, because of their sparsity. The pairs of words are mixed so that the patient will not obtain any clue from a consistent arrangement.

One-Syllable Pairs:

buck, rain	check, loves	cake, face
thin, pick	wolves, choked	cook, room
halves, stopped	chopped, lease	nice, tack

Multisyllable Pairs:

fulfill, checkers	unwise, static	tobacco, invasion
hasten, collect	spastic, mention	obstacle, souvenir
value, ticket	cessation, predicate	extricated, information
defect, hoarseness	relation, cosmetic	variation, constituted
ghetto, measure	scenery, departed	patriotic, nevertheless
jacket, social	property, easier	

"The following words have no plosive sounds. Let's pronounce them accurately, You may have to prolong the vibration longer than you have in the past. Sniff, inject and then say the word."

affiliation	effeminacy	harmonious	laziness
affluence	effluence	harness	leavening
aluminum	elevation	heavenly	linoleum
alveolar	evolutions	illumination	malformation
amaryllis	familiar	inanimation	marvelous
amazingly	generalize	inefficiency	meaningful
ammonium	generally	inflationism	militiaman
ammunition	half-hour	inherence	unusualness

Unit 26. Increasing Fluency Through Longer Phrases and Sentences

To the speech clinician: In order to obtain constant flow of phonation, it is necessary to improve the patient's ability to include longer and longer phrases in one air-charge. In addition to getting air in and out fast, the speaker must make only brief pauses between phrases (Snidecor). (Of course, pauses are also used for special purposes, such as for effect.) Phrases that are filled with plosives will be more easily pronounced and carried along. The phrases are presented in pairs. The first phrase will have plosive-laden words; the second will not. The patient will have to make full injections in the second phrase of each pair in order to maintain as much fluency as he obtained with the first phrase.

"I am going to give you two phrases. The first one may be easier than the second one because it has some plosive sounds. Try to say the second phrase with as much forward-flowing action as you use for the first phrase.

You must take in a good charge of air for it. It may be slightly harder, but the goal is to get good fluency throughout the phrase. Keep relaxed, don't strain and be sure to sniff before each phrase."

Two Syllables:

Come quick.	I'm fine.	too much	He will.
Beat it.	We are.	Watch it.	I know.
Get it.	They are.	Good night.	See him.
Bake it.	He says.	blue skies	He's fine.
Catch up.	I'm wrong.	Look out!	He's here.

Three Syllables:

Bring it back.	Follow me.	Jerk at it.	You seem fine.
Pick it up.	Are you there?	Take it up.	Where were you?
black and blue	He will know.	good as gold	I see him.
Hit it hard.	How are you?	Book it up.	I'm home now.
Jack's back aches.	Are you well?	spick and span	She was here.

Four Syllables:

What did it say?	Are you warm now?	Don't take a chance.	You knew him well?
Did Jack take it?	The house is fine.	It's not too late.	Where is he now?
Take it upstairs.	May I have more?	Dad was too tired.	I wish you well.
How'd you get it?	He has new shoes.	Take Tom to town.	He's easy now.
Tattle Tail Pat	Miss Ames was here.	Cut it to fit.	No one is in.

To the speech clinician: The following sentences and phrases may be dictated or the text may be given to the patient to read aloud. Instruct the patient to read them in order. Some of the sentences will require natural pauses between phrases.

"Read the following sentences and phrases."

To wit to wit towee.
I love Mother and Father.
Whither goest thou?
What a lovely living room.
When and why have you come?
I live to eat and eat to live.
We need a new safety slogan.

I will have mulligatawny soup.
Whatever you do, don't waste away your time.
The white whale whirled around the whaleboat.
His birthday is on the twenty-fifth day of the fifth month.

Let the apples ripen until they are big and red.
In olden times, beards were signs of wisdom.
Mother's cool, soft hand cooled the fevered brow.

Pretty Patty put her paddies in the pepper pot.
I am in the main room of the mansion.
I am sure I felt some rain on my face.
Visitation is very useful in our program.
Loving and living, working and loafing, saving and spending give zest to life.

"Repeat the following sets of phrases in order."

1. cookie jar
   chimney swift
   hickory tree bark
   home town celebrity
   negotiable instrument

2. butter dish
   shaving cream
   maple sugar candy
   champion footballer
   nontransferable docu-
       ment

3. tablecloth
   coffee grinder
   candy thermometer
   U.S. swimming
       champ
   sprawling metropolis

4. summer suit
   baby buggy
   pumpkin pie cutter
   German fried
       potatoes
   sadly deteriorated

5. onionskin
   football player
   broken-down old car
   celebrated astronaut
   maliciously and will-
       fully

6. spoon holder
   pigeon fancier
   Jack the Jumping Jack
   perforated ulcer
   fully recompensated

7. yard master
   dinner table
   chocolate cake
   substantially correct
   unexplained
       obstinacy

8. pageboy bob
   ticket taker
   comptometer
       operator
   accommodation
       paper
   fiduciary officer

9. milk pitcher
   time to go now
   bookkeeping machine
   tremendous oppor-
       tunity
   zealous administrator

"Use the following sentence to increase the number of words per air-charge:

I am going downtown tonight at six o'clock on the bus to buy a new suit.

Endeavor to increase the amount of air you take in but without straining. Then endeavor to prolong the voiced sound as long as you feel you have air to maintain it. Do this exercise many times at home not only for increasing air-charge but for proper phrasing.

"Start counting with 21 (three syllables) and extend your production per air-charge to 22 and 23. That would equal nine syllables. Perhaps you can add another number because all of these have plosive syllables. Work on this many times during the day."

To the speech clinician: At this point, give Periodic Test 5 (page 98).

Unit 27. Improving Fluency by Blending Syllables

To the speech clinician: In fluent speech, the speaker does not keep syllables precisely intact as they are spelled and separated in the dictionary. They are blended in a natural manner for an easy flow of phonation; that is, a consonant at the end of one syllable may be joined to the initial vowel of the syllable that follows. This technique is doubly helpful if the blended consonant happens to be a plosive, which may contribute somewhat to the production of the following vowel. The speaker may not be aware that he does not have to work as hard on pronouncing the following vowel as he does when the vowel is in the initial position of a word.

"Did you have a lot of fun working on the sentence about going downtown to buy a suit? ... Let's hear how many syllables you can get on the first air-charge. ... You tried too hard. Don't keep on trying when you don't have air left. Take it easy, sniff before you start. Try it again. ... You got seven syllables. That's a good start right now, for your period of training. But keep on working.

"Today, we are going to help you get even more forward-flowing speech by joining the final syllable of a word to the beginning of the second syllable. Say *kup.* ... Now say *spea-kup.* ... You really said *speak up.*[1] ... How would you say *back of?* ... You put the /k/ with the *of,* so it comes out *bac-kof.* Here is another one; say *putting.* ... You have to separate the two /t/'s, so it comes out with one /t/ at the end of the first syllable and the other /t/ at the beginning of the second syllable. You pronounce only the last /t/. Try it: *put-ting.* ... Try *climbing.* ... That's right; you emphasize the /m/ with the second syllable. How about *aiming.* ... Again the /m/ goes with the last syllable: *ai-ming.* ... Say *going.* ... You have to put a /w/ in front of the *ing* when you make the sound real fast, the lips moving from the vowel to the /ŋ/. So pronounce it as *go-wing.* ... That's good. Try *swar-ming.* ... Say *starting.* ... That's right; the /t/ goes with the second syllable. Here's a good sentence for you. Say this: *Jac-kand-Jill.* ... *wen-*

---

[1] Write demonstration words on a blackboard or on paper, showing the proper way of blending.

tup the hill. ... to-ge-ta-pai-lof-wa-ter. ... Now say it quickly and hear if you don't really say the blends that way. ... Here is another sentence: *Hel-p(h)im ge-t(h)is coa-ton.* ... Say it again very quickly and hear how you say those final syllables. ... You should be able to take this list of words[2] and work out the pronunciation and blends before you look at the correct answer.[3]

[2] Cover up the second line of each group of words with a card. Have the patient look at the first line and say the words with what he thinks is the correct blend; then have him check himself on the second line.

spinning	*swimming*
(spin-ning)	*(swim-ming)*
taking	*coming*
(ta-king)	*(co-ming)*
watching	*during*
(wat-ching)	*(du-ring)*
rumbling	*rolling*
(rum-bling)	*(rol-ling)*
blowing	*wearing*
(blo-wing)	*(wea-ring)*
hammer	*boating*
(ham-mer)	*(boa-ting)*
burning	*walking*
(bur-ning)	*(wa[l]-king)*
baking	*bring it along*
(ba-king)	*(bri-ngi-ta-long)*
hang it up	*set it up*
(ha-ngi-tup)	*(se-ti-tup)*
back up	*closer*
(bac-kup)	*(clo-ser)*
quicken	*whiten*
(quic-ken)	*(whi-ten)*
going	*fix it*
(go-wing)	*(fik-sit)*
put it in	*aiming*
(pu-ti-tin)	*(ai-ming)*
black and white	*swarming*
(bla-kand-white)	*(swar-ming)*
Want to light up?	*climbing*
(Wan-ta-ligh-tup?)	*(cli-m[b]ing)*

Find other words and put them in sentences, dividing their syllables as directed above.

[3] For additional information on blending, consult Hahn *et al.;* Hyman (1960); and Peacher.

Unit 28. Improving Fluency Through Rate of Speaking

If the patient has consistently and faithfully mastered the techniques that have been presented up to this point, he should now be ready to demonstrate how nearly adequate his rate of speaking is, that is, for esophageal speakers. We have worked on fast air intake and fast air outgo, and on increasing the number of syllables produced for each air-charge while at the same time sustaining a steady flow of esophageal vibration.

Snidecor set up a table for a given passage in which he suggested that sixty to seventy-two words would be regarded as adequate, eighty to ninety as good and rates up to 120 as excellent. It would appear that the laryngectomee should be able to produce one word per second, which would be adequate at this stage of learning. Therefore, we have prepared some simple tests (in addition to the Periodic Tests) to evaluate the progress toward fluency the laryngectomee has achieved. These tests should be repeated many times to improve skills.

Test A is simply a test of the number of digits that the patient can count in one air-charge. He is asked to count as far as he can after one air intake and then stop. Superior speakers count within a range of four to ten numbers (eleven syllables), with an average of six in one air-charge (Snidecor). Normal speakers are reported to be able to reach 40, but we have had several swimmers and users of musical wind instruments who reached as high as 60.

Test B is designed to test the same ability but with the use of multi-syllable numbers with plosive consonants, such as 22, which will permit a slightly faster rate. The patient is asked to count as far as he can on one air-charge, beginning at 22. In tests A and B, it should be impressed on the patient that he must not inject again during the test, but rather must stop at once if he does inject a second time.

Test C is a simple effort on the part of the laryngectomee to read as many words as he can in a single air-charge.

Test D is more difficult because the patient is asked to read prose for one minute and then count the number of words read. This test will indicate how consistently he makes air-charges and sustains them for a continuous flow of sound.

Test A

Instruction to speaker: "I am going to ask you to start counting from 1 up. Make one injection of air and start counting until the air is gone. If you try to inject air again after you start, stop at once. Start when I say 'Go!' When you finish, tell me the last number you spoke clearly. Ready? Go!" (If 7 is reached, count this as two syllables.)

Test B

Instruction to speaker: "Start at 22 and count as long as you can with one good air-charge. Stop if you try to inject again. Tell me what number you spoke last. Ready? Go!

Test C

Instruction to speaker: "Here is a sentence for you to read. *Now is the time for all good men to come to the aid of their party.* When I say 'Go,' take in a good air-charge and start reading. Stop when you can't make any more sound or if you try to take in a second air-charge. Tell me the last word you were able to produce well. Here is the sentence. Ready? Go!"

Test D

Instruction to speaker: "Here is a paragraph that has been used in research to study various aspects of speech. I wish to find out how many words you can read in one minute. Read without hurrying, and try to pronounce each word clearly. Read to make yourself understood. Start reading when I say 'Go' and stop reading when I say 'Stop.' Mark a line through the word you last spoke clearly. Get ready. Go!"

Once there was a young rat named Arthur who could [10] never make up his mind. Whenever the other rats asked [20] him if he would like to go out with them, [30] he would answer, "I don't know." And when they said, [40] "Would you like to stay at home?" he wouldn't say [50] yes or no either. He would always shirk at making [60] a choice.

One day his aunt said to him, "Now [70] look here. No one will ever care for you if [80] you carry on like this; you have no more mind [90] than a blade of grass." The young rat coughed and [100] looked wise as usual, but said nothing. "Don't you think [110] so?" asked his aunt, stamping with her foot, for she [120] couldn't bear to see the young rat so cold-blooded. [130] "I don't know" was all the young rat ever answered. [140] And then he would walk off and think for an [150] hour whether he should stay in his hole in the ground [160] or go out and walk.

Phase V. Restoring Melody in the Laryngectomee's Voice

The most common impression auditors obtain from hearing a laryngectomee speak is the roughness or hoarseness of the voice. Several factors are responsible for this. The normal firm support of the air column for voiceless consonants and for activation of the vocal folds, and the inherent effect of the weight, volume and flexibility of the vocal folds are missing in the laryngectomee (Nichols). Likewise, the production of air vibrated by the much less efficient esophagus and the neoglottis, flowing forward through the resonance chambers, loses the brilliance and certain musical aspects that are present in the laryngeal voice. The result is hoarseness, monotony and lack of expression.

The question is asked: To what extent can the voice of the laryngectomized person be improved? If we consider the natural musical aspect of the normal voice, we know that it comes from the vowels, not from the consonants. If the vowels are well resonated and articulated, the quality of the voice will be more likely to please the listener. Likewise, duration of utterance is an outstanding difference between spoken and sung vowels. In speech the vibrations of the vowel, as recorded on a smoked drum, would cover a very short span of space compared with the extended recording of vibrations from the sung vowel. Vowels may be prolonged or shortened in speech to meet the purpose of the speaker, just as they are by singers to meet the requirements of the composer who wishes to create a particular effect. In the same way, words are spoken normally at varying pitches and intensities, whereas the laryngectomee, who does not vary greatly the pitch and/or loudness in his conversation, will display unattractive monotony. Finally, the basic pitch (average conversational) level of the laryngectomee's voice is usually much lower than the preoperative pitch level. This and other characteristics of his voice cause considerable embarrassment to the patient. Therefore, quality and pitch (with loudness related) must be included in any plan for developing melody in the voice of the laryngectomized person. Hence, it is desirable that the characteristics which are present in a melodic voice should be present to some degree in the speaking voice of the laryngectomee.

Perhaps we are arguing too finely or too strenuously on the subject of melody for the voice of a laryngectomee. After all, the laryngectomee may not have had a melodious voice before surgery. Some patients may object to efforts to give them what they may regard as the language of kings. Unfortunately, too, we will not always have an opportunity to put our ideals into practice because some patients withdraw from instruction far too early. Perhaps, then, we can only set up some instructions that we consider will be helpful in making the voices of laryngectomees more attractive to their auditors. We can, at least, inform them of the possibilities for improving their speech, and let them decide for themselves how to use them.

Unit 29. Expanding the Pitch Range

"The average male esophageal speaker has a pitch level during conversational speech that is one octave lower than that of the person with a normal larynx.[1] Let's first find out how much range in pitch you have. We have surprised speakers who did not realize that they used more than one pitch. We know of speakers who

[1] Damsté; Diedrich and Youngstrom; Snidecor.

have a full octave range. One cowboy can sing his range songs almost as well as he did before laryngectomy. A 12-year-old boy can sing a full octave. If you can increase your pitch range—that is, the lowest note and the highest note that you can make—and express words at varying pitches, you will make your voice much more attractive.

"You have heard people say *ha, haaaa!*[2] when they surprised someone. The second *hah* was spoken at a much higher pitch. Try it. ... Your second *hah* was noticeably higher than the speaking pitch you are using. It was also louder. Let's try three pitches. Use *bah* and go up three steps like this,[3] as in *do, re, me.* ... That was easy.[4] Next time, we will go up three steps and down again to *do. It's do, re, me, re, do.* Use *bah* again.[5] ... You did quite well. You didn't know you had so much music available in your voice. That's going to be helpful. Let's go a little higher; go up four notes. That will be *do, re, me, fa, sol.* Use *bah* again.[6] ... You didn't have enough air support for that highest note. It may be your limit, too. This exercise can be done many times a day. Try it once more. Take a good breath and tense your abdomen to support it. ... Let's try another trick. You have heard the tune "Three Blind Mice"?[7] Hit the highest note on *three* at *me* on the scale and come down to *re, do* with *blind mice.* ... You have proved to yourself that you have almost half of an octave. Do that exercise many times. Hum songs like "America"; hum hymns and your favorite songs.[8] We can use those pitches to improve your ability to express yourself for certain meanings."

Unit 30. Improving Voice Through Inflection

"Now you have an opportunity to put expression in the voice by using a variation in pitch. One way to put music in your voice is when you say very simple things such as a greeting. You've

　　　　haaaa!
[2] *ha*

　　　　　bah　　　　(*mi*)
　　　　bah　　　　(*re*)
[3] *bah*　　　　(*do*)

[4] It is expected that the patient may strain or stretch his neck to reach his higher notes. He may also lift his chin. Let him experiment.

　　　　　bah
　　　　bah　　*bah*
[5] *bah*　　　　　*bah*

　　　　　　bah　(sol)
　　　　　bah　(fa)
　　　　bah　(mi)
　　　bah　(re)
[6] *bah*　(do)

[7] *Three*　　(me)
　　blind　　(re)
　　　mice　(do)

[8] Consult M.C.L. Greene, and Hodson and Oswald, for more information on musical activities. The latter authors advocate extensive exercises in humming.

heard friends greet you with a lilt in *Hello*. Say it like this.[1] ... Try putting music in your greeting. ... That's what we call inflection. You may glide upward and downward, depending on the effect you wish to make or merely on your emotional response to something that happens. When you question a person's remarks, you say *Yes* with a rising note.[2] ... Try it. ... Good. Suppose that someone tells you about an accident. You might say: *Oh, no-oo.*[3] ... Here's another greeting. Say *How are you?* on the tune *do me do.*[4] ... A hearty greeting, it might have a long *ahre* before you come down. Try *How ahahahre you?*[5] ... Or, you might say: *How do you doooo-oo?*[6] Here is another one. You are surprised when someone accuses you. You go up on *me*.[7] Say *I am so sorry for her*, by inflecting on *sorry*.[8] ... Practice greeting your friends with a *Hi*,[9] inflecting up and down. ... I would suggest you hum or say *do, re, me, me, re, do* many times a day.[10]

"We don't intend for you to sing but to vary the pitch of your voice and inflect when you want to show your feelings. People will comment that you talk almost as you did before surgery.[11] Practice inflections in these phrases. The accented word is to be given a higher pitch. Try *It's my' turn*. ... *I don't like' that*. ... Good. When you talk, raising your eyebrows with your inflection will help people to understand from your facial expression. Practice

                    looo
[1] *He   oo.*

              es?
[2] *Ye*

[3] *Oh no*
              oo.

                        are (me)
[4] *How (do)   you? (do)*

              ahahahre
[5] *How   you?*

                      doooo
[6] *How do you   oo?*

              eeee?
[7] *Me*

              so sor
                    ry for
[8] *I am   her!*

[9] *Hi*
        eeeeee.

                  me
            re   re
[10] *Do   do*

                    tum
                tum   tum
              tum   tum

[11] Use discretion with your suggestions; some people will never regain a "lovely" voice, such as a female laryngectomee might wish to have.

these sentences with marked inflections.[12] Make up some that you can use at home."

[12] Put a lilt in the accented word or syllable, that is, inflect it upward:

It's my' turn; I don't like' that; I don't like that'; What a lovely' day; What time' are you go'-ing? Isn't it time' to leave'? Now' what do you want? What do you want now'? Will you have a sandwich'? Yes', thank you; You're wel'-come; That's wonder'-ful.

Unit 31. Raising the Speaking Level of the Voice

"Now that we have practiced at higher pitches, and have found that it is possible to speak at different pitch levels, it should be interesting to try to raise the pitch level of your speaking voice. You know that your voice is an octave lower than it was before surgery, and that you have been speaking in a monotonous tone. Your voice may be more attractive if you speak at a higher pitch most of the time. One method of improving the voice is to intone at a higher pitch level until you become familiar with it and retain it in your auditory memory. Try this one. Say *Today is Tuesday.*[1] ... You said the words at the same pitch. Raise the pitch a note higher for each word, as in *do, re, me.* ... Good. Say it again but after intoning *Tuesday*, keep intoning the word at that level.[2] ... Next, go up again, but after saying *Tuesday* at the upper pitch, count *one, two, three, four, five*, all at the upper pitch.[3] ... Nice! You can do the same with any words, but to practice you might use the days of the week. By intoning at the upper level, you develop a better voice up there and at the same time begin to feel that it can be habitual.

"You get a special dividend by talking at that higher level. You discover that you can inflect still higher, at a level that you first are not able to reach. So, let's work on it this way.

```
                      Tuesday.   (me)
               is    (re)
[1] Today      (do)
```

```
                   Tuesday, Tuesday.
            is
[2] Today
```

```
         is Tuesday one two three...
[3] Today
```

Say the phrase *Today is Tuesday,* with Tuesday at the upper level; then say *How are you?* with the inflection still higher.[4] ... Do you understand how to practice this new speaking level? You first have to drill until it's habitual and then inflect from there. Another way to get started is to intone *do, re, me* and begin talking at the level of *me.* ... Try this: *do, re, me, nice day today.*[5] ... But keep the sentence at the new pitch. You may even inflect the word *day.*[6] Once more. ... That's much better. The thing to do is to read sentences and paragraphs at the new pitch level. You may start a paragraph with *do, re, me. Once upon a time,* etc. Or you can sit at the piano or use a pitch pipe to blow the note that you are to use as your speaking pitch level.[7] If you want to make a speech you do the same thing, sitting there and tapping the note occasionally. Then you must learn to speak to your family at the higher pitch."

$$\text{[4] Today is Tuesday, How } \overset{are}{} \text{ you?}$$

$$\text{[5] Do } \overset{re}{} \text{ me. Nice day today.}$$

$$\text{[6] Do } \overset{re}{} \text{ me. Nice } \overset{day}{} \text{ today.}$$

[7] First find the note on the piano that matches your present pitch level. Then go up two notes and intone at that level until it becomes habitual. Of course, the rise of the level two tones is subject to trial and error by the therapist and the patient.

To the speech clinician: At this point, give Periodic Test 6 (page 98).

Phase VI. Increasing the Intelligibility of the Laryngectomee's Speech

Many teachers accept the quality of laryngectomees' voices as an inevitable, unchanging aspect. With the pitch of the male voice lowered one octave below the natural pitch level, and the female voice sounding like a male voice, there appears to be limited opportunity to improve the voice. But this is not entirely true. Exercises have already been used to improve the quality of the voice. Now it is desirable that time be spent on improving other aspects of speech, such as intelligibility (DiCarlo *et al.*)—that is, the articulation of the vowels and consonants. The purity of the vowels may be improved also by more accurate use of the articulators in adjusting the oral cavities for their production (V. Anderson; Hanley and Thurman; Snidecor). The adjustments must be made with sufficient accuracy to differentiate each vowel and consonant from the others, and to render the unvoiced consonants more audible. Relaxation of the neck, pharyngeal, oral and facial structures as well as sufficient, steady support of the diaphragm are contributing factors to clarity and to differentiating one sound from another.

Since the laryngectomee has made considerable progress to have reached the present stage of therapy, there now remain opportunities (a) to make marked improvement in articulating vowels, and (b) to improve the ability to differentiate similar words.

Unit 32. Improving the Quality of Voiced Sounds: Vowels

"Your speech will be more pleasant and more easily understood if you work intensively on the vowels and consonants. Say these pairs of vowels in one air-charge and make each vowel distinctly different and slightly prolonged.[1] Listen for the differences in the sound and feel the differences in the muscular actions. Sniff and say *peat-pot.* ... The first vowel was long with a smile on the lips; the second vowel was short and was made after lowering the jaw. Observe things like these. Again: *peat-pot.* ... That was much clearer. Do the pair five times while watching yourself in this mirror. Hold it and watch your lips move rapidly from one position to the other. Exaggerate the movements. Get the tongue up for a final /t/. ... Those were much better than the first ones. Did you see the differences in the mirror and feel the differences in the muscular action? ... Good. People will understand you better. Here is another pair. Say *cat-cool.* ... In the first word, the jaw is down, the lips are broadened; in the second, the jaw is up and the lips are protruded and rounded. Say *cat-cool* five times; watch in the mirror. ... Much clearer. Do the other words on the list the same way; exaggerate to get good muscle feeling and hearing of the sound.

"Here are some double vowels; we call them diphthongs. Hear the two vowels as you glide from one to the other. Make a positive change in the lips, jaw or tongue as you glide. Feel the gliding action. First say *ah-ee.* ... Say it again faster. ... It sounds almost as one because of the gliding action. Let's say *pie.* ... End the vowel with a quick, brief smile for the *ee.* Once more, *pie.* For the word *cow* say *ah-oo.* ... Now *cah-oo.* ... Say it quickly. ... Blend and prolong the

[1] *peat-pot; cat-cool; pit-ball; put-pot; cop-cape; good-cot; took-take; cool-keel; peg-pig; bell-bill; did-deed; beat-boot; big-bug; gill-gull; comb-come; let-late; tell-tale; met-meet; aim-am; all-old; egg-nog; itch-age; oaf-I've; sot-sought; don-dawn; cod-cawed; hock-hawk; frame-from; bar-bore; cart-court; farm-form; par-pour; coal-call; pole-pall; bowl-ball; cut-caught; buck-balk; dun-din; down-dun; doom-dome; full-fool; stood-stewed; should-shoved; wood-wooed; feud-food; cute-coat; cue-coo; tuck-took; look-foot; dock-duck; pop-pup; pot-putt; pout-pert, head-heard; port-pert.*

vowels in *boy.* ... Do the same for the next words. Say *toe.* ... *cowboy.* ... *key chain.* ... *turtle dove.* ... *ten-day furlough.* ... From now on, read paragraphs aloud and prolong or exaggerate the diphthongs you observe."[2]

[2] Words to practice to articulate clearly double vowels, (dipthongs):

cow; plow; how; bough; about; lout; shy; my; wry; lie; guy; vie; boy; joy; coy; annoy; toy; Floy; join; pay; bee; Jay; Kay; Wray; way; nay; toe; roe; foe; boat; coat; nose.

We may have peas soon; How high is his balloon? Go out and hoe the rows of peas and beans; No more does the plowman say; "Gee and Haw" to his plodding team; The machine has replaced the team; Don't you know what to do? Fix it now; A stitch in time saves nine; Count your blessings.

Unit 33. Improving the Quality of Voiced Sounds: Consonants

"Laryngectomees may not pronounce clearly the final consonant of a word, the final syllable of a word or the final word of a phrase or sentence.[1] In our clinical experience, we have observed especially that the voiced consonants in the final position are not pronounced clearly. The tongue may take the approximate position for the sound but the voiced aspect may not be heard. Say the word *cabs.* ... Do you believe you produced a clear-cut /z/? ... I didn't hear it. This time, finish the word by holding /z/ longer: *cabzzzzzz.* ... That was hard to do. You must get enough air in to produce two voiced sounds and the voiced aspect of /s/. Be sure that you feel and hear the vibration to the very end of the word. People will not understand you easily if you don't finish the final sounds. They will ask you to repeat your word so say *cubs.* ... You made an /s/ sound but there was no voice. Hold the vibrations from below long enough to carry them through the /z/ sound.

[1] See Diedrich and Youngstrom's summary of the difficulties with sounds among laryngectomees as found by the researches of J.O. Anderson; DiCarlo *et al.;* and Hyman.

Again: *cubs*. ... Try *floodzzzz*. ... *sisterszzzz*. ... *singers*. ... *comedies*. ... Buzz all of the final /s/ sounds: Say *Two sisters were stars in the comedies*. ... Those were much more distinct. Here are more words for you to practice on.[2]

"Final /d/ is another typical problem. Say *child*. ... I heard *chile*. Carry the vibration through the /d/. Try it again. ... That was more like it, but it was not distinct. Let's add something to the word for practice. Say *childuh*. ... You got the tongue up for the /d/ and held the vibration longer. Now say *child*. ... No final /d/! So you must practice adding the extra sound to the final /d/ or /b/ or similar sounds. Say *colduh*. ... Now, *cold*. ... Try *headuh*. ... Now *head*. ... You are getting better final voicing. Work on this word list[3] and make sure you hear and feel the final voiced action in every word. Make up sentences ending in /d/.

"Final words and sounds are not heard when you haven't enough vibrated air left in your esophagus. That means you have to learn to retain enough air in it for the final sound, if it is voiced. Here are some /b/ final sounds. Try *sobuh*. ... Now *sob*. ... *rib*. ... *robe*. ... Think of the extra, prolonged sound so you carry the vibration through it. Try *cobuh-cob*. ... *Bobuh*. ... *sub*. ... *rub*. ... Work on the list[4] and make up additional words to use in sentences..

[2] Words ending in /z/ but with the voiced aspect prominently produced in order to be heard:

webs; pans; tubs; horns; robs; rains; tolls; signs; girls; dolls; storms; farms; robes; drums; halls; clothes; truths; gives; leaves.

Mothers smooth the pains of boys and girls in their homes; Nature gives leaves to the trees in the spring; Buds on the red buds swelled and burst into red.

[3] Have the patient first add the vowel /ʌ/ (*uh*) to the final d, b, j, and g, then say the final sound clearly without the added sound:

golduh-gold;   holduh-hold; tolduh-told;   crieduh-cried; used; raised; praised; buzzed; Fold and mold the rolled gold; Load it in the second hold. Today is Dad's birthday.

ride; hand; head; good; did; made; mud; flood; could; hid; bed; bid; need; made; land; hand; band; bud; kind; find; send; lend; bird; bide; side; rid; red; rained; bind; faded; readied; blinded; sided;

[4] *Bobuh-Bob;   sobuh-sob; rubuh-rub; knob; job; rob; fib; web; crab; grab; robe; globe; cube; crib; scrub; web; tube; robbed; robed; tub; knob; cub; bribe; cab; tube; job; jab; ribbed; robed.*

Why does Bob hobnob with the mob? Redbird, blackbird, bluebird; keep a tab on them all.

"The same problem applies to final /g/ and final /dʒ/ (j). Say *egguh. ... beguh. ... leguh. ... egg. ... beg. ... leg. ...* Those are better than when we started a half-hour ago on voiced endings.[5] Let's hear what you do with the final /dʒ/. Say *judgeuh. ... pageuh. ... cageuh. ... largeuh. ... judge. ... page. ... cage. ... large. ...* Work on the word list and put the words in sentences.[6] Hear and feel the vibration on the final sounds.

"Many times a speaker will bring his tongue up for the final /l/ sound but will not voice it. Let's try something. First say the word *baw. ...* Now change that to *ball. ...* Your tongue was flat for *baw*, and the tip went up to the dental ridge for the /l/. But I didn't hear the sound of /l/. Practice this: *all, all, ball. ...* Hold the /l/ a little longer as the sound of the bell lingers when it is tolled. Say *ell-ell-belllll. ...* Hold the tongue in place and feel the vibration passing around its tip. That makes the /l/ sound. Roll out the /l/ sounds on these: *roll. ... toll. ... will. ...* Put the /l/ in a sentence: *Will William get his fill of the pill? ... Fill the pail full. ... Bill took a bill from the till. ...* Linger with the /l/'s on the list of words.[7]

"Here is another sound that is not spoken well at the end, the sound of /r/. We have to do the same as we did with the other sounds and hold the voice longer. But to get a good idea of how to do it, we will start with a word that begins with /r/, *ride*. We start with a vowel *ah* and curl our tongue up for /r/, so it sounds like *ah-ir*. Say it this way: *ah-ir-run, run. ah-ir-ride. ...* Now let's change the vowel part to the end of the word like this: *fear-ir. ...* Hold the voice right to the end. *fear-ir. ...* Now say *fear-ir, fear. ... sir-ir-sir, sir. ... pear-ir-pear, pear. ...* Fine. Say *tear. ... wear. ... rear. ... seer. ... sure. ... fir. ... I fear the horse will rear up. ... The bumper was torn when the car was hit from the rear. ... The roar of the racing car hurt*

[5] *egguh-egg;   diguh-dig; biguh-big; buguh-bug; tug; lug; frog; hug; leg; beg; pig; dog; hog; fog; frog; rug; tug; pug; bug; dug.*

Tag the log for the next tugboat; The dog bit Pegleg's pegleg; The frog in the bog sought the bogbug.

Have the patient make up sentences for the other words.

[6] *ageuh-age;   pageuh-page; judgeuh-judge;   bridgeuh-bridge; sludge; fudge; college; large; edge; rage; badge; cage; orange; huge; hedge; image; carriage; wage; oblige; ridge; lodge; forge; gorge.*

[7] *all; ball; call; fall; tall; tell; well; will; fill; mill; hill; soil; toil; file; tile; rile; wile; rail; foil; coil; fail; mail; tale; kale; sail; mall; sell; fell; bell; yell; well; teal; peal; wheel; feel; deal; heel; ill.*

He will fulfill the pledge that Will willed in his will; The steel mill paid the bill in full; Out on bail, he stole the US mail; When he pulled the bell rope, he fell to the floor; A smile will bring you a smile in return; Lill spilled the milk when she slipped and fell on the mall; Bill took the doll away from Jill; Will paid the doctor his bill after being ill.

his ear. ... From now on, end the /r/ words with a burr."[8]

[8] The /r/ should have a "burr" in front and at the end of words:

ring; rich; river; ribbon; rock; robber; rug; rub; room; roar; rise; ripe; rear; rare; fair; chair; hair; care; bear; peer; pear; order; four; roses; four-year-old daughter; Read as you run; Rob rang the dinner bell; Father bought mother a dinner platter; The railroad runs on steel rails; Bill took cash from the till; The bumper was torn when the car was hit from the rear; The roar of the car was hard on the ear.

Unit 34. Differentiating Similar Words

"One of the reasons for misunderstanding laryngectomees is that voiced and unvoiced sounds are not properly differentiated.[1] For example, *ice* and *eyes* may sound alike to some people if they do not hear well enough to discriminate between them, or if the speaker does not pronounce the words differently or the speech is given in an unfavorable environment. I will cover up my face so that you cannot see my lips when I say these two sentences. The first sentence is *Let him dry it out.* What did I say? ... I will say a similar sentence: *Let him try it out. What did I say?* ... You got them correctly. I articulated too well. Let's reverse things. You say the sentence to me and I will tell you what I heard. What's the first one? ... *What size of bill was it?* Was that right? ... Oh, you said *pill.* Try another. ... You said *What a lovely peach.* Was I right? ... Oh, you said *What a lovely beach.* Maybe I don't hear well but it does prove that you did not articulate them well enough. Take these sentences and say them to a relative or friend, but cover your mouth with a paper so that they can't read your lips. Then ask them to say back the sentence. It will show you how well you articulate."

[1] The patient should have someone repeat these sentences after him in order to hear how well he pronounces similar-sounding words. He should say each sentence once with each of the alternate words:

a. *Let him* dry (try) *it out.*
b. *What size of* bill (pill) *was it?*
c. *He kept on* riding (writing).
d. *What a lovely* beach (peach).
e. *When did you get the* coat (goat)?
f. *The yardman fought a young* bear (mare).
g. *I saw him in the* boat (moat).
h. *The officer sent out a* card (guard).
i. *I'll get in* touch (dutch).
j. *The company will fix the* gable (cable).
k. *I intend to take a quick* bath (path).

This is a good exercise for groups. Have one laryngectomee read the sentences with his lips concealed. For more fun, make up more sentences like these.

Phase VII. Increasing the Loudness of the Laryngectomee's Voice

Little concern is given to the loudness of the laryngectomee's voice during his early efforts to talk. He first has to make many other psychophysiological adjustments to his altered voice mechanism in order to regain a voice. Furthermore, we have asked the laryngectomee to take it easy, to relax, not to strain in his efforts to produce an esophageal sound. Our first goal was to get a good voice by whatever method we could. Now that he has learned to speak with a fairly even, uninterrupted flow of phonation, he should be ready to render his speaking more understandable and more acceptable to his auditors.

Among the abilities the patient should have acquired is supportive breathing and its coordination with phonation. This is the basic vehicle for acquiring adequate loudness or volume (van den Berg *et al.;* M.C.L. Greene; Hodson and Oswald). But such a demand calls upon the breathing musculature to work harder, and he does not have the adjustment capacity that is obtainable through the great pneumolaryngeal power of the normal speaker. All that he can do is force esophageal air out of the neoglottis with whatever increased power he can engender (Strother). Even then the laryngectomee may be subject to muscle tensions that defeat his efforts or affect the quality of his voice. (Generaux). Hence, if supportive breathing has not been adequately developed by this time, time must be taken out to do it. (For a thorough discussion of loudness in a laryngectomee, see Snidecor 1968.) A review of the early units of instruction should be given. However, numerous methods are available for improving the loudness of the laryngectomee's speaking voice, including the following:

1. The simplest procedure to develop loudness is to have the patient practice reading or speaking at levels of slightly increasing loudness, provided he does it without developing tensions in the speech mechanism. When he becomes adjusted to the new level of amplified voice he should endeavor to make it as melodious as it was at the lower level.

2. Certain adjustments of the speech mechanism may enable the patient to improve the loudness of his voice. Moving the head to different positions while talking may reveal to the speaker one particular position that enables him to produce a louder voice (Moore). The physiological effect may be a slight alteration of the neoglottis or the neoglottic air chamber (esophagus) (Snidecor). We have seen an occasional patient who always talked with his head held to one side. When asked why he did it, he replied that he got a louder voice. Another person held his hand on his chest as if he were saluting the flag or had a pain. If he withdrew his hand, his voice faded. In these cases, the fixed positions, necessary for adequate loudness, may be eliminated by gradually releasing pressure or slowly changing the position while prolonging vowel sounds or phrases. Knepflar states that such maneuvers may eventually produce a louder voice with the head in a natural position. Use of an amplifier and headphones or of the TOK-BAK device is helpful in monitoring the change in loudness.

3. Another person may talk while he pinches his neck just above the stoma in order to maintain adequate loudness. McClear and other staff members of the IAL voice institutes have demonstrated this technique. The patient is requested to inject and phonate as he applies the pressure. If he obtains a louder sound, the instructor requests him to prolong it while the pressure is slowly released. Other patients were persuaded to wear a

small square of sponge rubber pressed tightly against the above-mentioned area in order to maintain a suitable loudness. Later efforts were then made to produce the same loudness without the rubber.

4. Systematic practice in developing kinesthetic awareness and auditory awareness may help the patient to retain increased loudness. For example, the patient is requested to read in a soundproof room while white noise is slowly increased in intensity. At a given level, the noise is cut off, but the patient is requested to continue his reading at the newly attained degree of loudness. His attention is called to the kinesthetic stimuli as well as to the auditory feedback which may enable him to retain the louder voice for conversational use. Another technique is to use an amplifier and headphones. The patient reads continuously, speaking into the microphone, while a masking sound is introduced through the headphones. During this procedure, the patient's amplified voice is being recorded. Later, the patient plays back the voice and tries to match the loudness level as he rereads the passage. The procedure may be altered simply by placing safety plugs in the ears while the voice is being recorded, provided the person has good hearing.

Another method of training the patient to use increased loudness is to conduct a conversation in a soundroom into which is sent a noise level equivalent to factory noise (about 90 dB). The patient is requested to notice kinesthetic cues that he may retain later on in order to adapt himself to the new level. Throughout all of these procedures, tension and strain must be avoided. Furthermore, adequate abdominal support must be developed for the newly adapted loudness. This technique has been quite successful with dysphonic laryngeal patients who work in noisy places.

5. Emotionally laden words and phrases are also helpful in demonstrating adequate loudness of esophageal voice (Snidecor 1968). Snidecor tells of one patient who wished to call quickly to someone at a distance. He simply inhaled more deeply and stuck out his chin to make a much louder voice. Words such as *STOP it! No, NO! Don't DO that! OH, No!* and *WOW!* may be practiced. Patients often are startled when they hear themselves talking more loudly. However, in using these devices, we should always maintain as easy a functioning of the speech mechanism as we can. Otherwise, the product may be undesirable in quality. In making these calls, the patient is often urged to sing out the words to insure greater ease of production. This idea is extremely helpful to persons giving orders in noisy places.

6. Monotony of speaking pitch level and loudness may also be altered by taking advantage of accents on certain syllables and by placing emphasis on certain words (stress). These will now be demonstrated.

Unit 35. Using Loudness for Accent

"Here are some words that have one syllable accented, that is, it is spoken more loudly than the other syllables. In these words, the syllable to be accented determines the meaning. For example, the word *PRO-ject* means something to be done, but *pro-JECT* means to extend or send forward. Let's try *PRO-ject*. ... The other: *pro-JECT*. ... Try this: *pro-DUCE*. ... Now: *PRO-duce*. ... Remember; don't strain. You really just make them a bit louder, so it is not a struggle to do that much, but it improves understanding of your conversation. Let's try some three-syllable words, one of whose syllables is to be accented. Try *COM-pe-tent*. ... *com-PAN-ion*. ... Here are two four-syllable words: *el-e-VA-tion*. ... *el-e-MENT-al*. ... Here's a list of words to practice on. Be sure to emphasize or accent the right syllable."[1]

[1] *TEN-der; TEM-per; pre-PARE; TEN-nis; sup-PLY; con-TENT; CON-tract; con-TRACT; RE-cord; re-CORD; SUB-ject; sub-JECT; PRO-ject; pro-JECT; PRO-duce; pro-DUCE; te-LEG-ra-phy; pre-SENT; PRE-sent; SUS-pect; sus-PECT; POP-u-lar; SIM-u-late; SKEP-ti-cal; EL-e-vate; el-e-VA-tion.*

The patient should look up two-syllable words which have different meanings depending on the accent, and multi-syllable words that may have a major and minor accent.

Unit 36. Using Loudness for Stress (Emphasis)

"Another method of using loudness is to emphasize an entire word in a phrase or an entire phrase in a sentence.[1] This is called *stress*. Just say simply without any meaning to it the sentence: *I am mad*. ... It doesn't sound as if the speaker means anything. Now, say it this way: *I am MAD*. ... You know how the speaker feels. Say it again that way. ... Let's change the idea to a matter of doubt. *I AM mad*. ... A boy might brag about his father: *MY father is BIGGER than YOURS*. ... Say this: *NOW is the time*. ... *for ALL GOOD MEN*. ... *to come to the AID*. ... *of the PARTY*. ... Now say the entire sentence and emphasize the words that you think are important. ... You might say that sentence many times during the day. Change it by em-

[1] The emphasized words are written in capital letters:

Come to ME; COME to me; Don't DO that; Don't do THAT; Easy COME, easy GO; Are you happy with your new JOB? I had a GOOD TIME last night; I had a good time LAST night; I tell you RIGHT NOW, gentlemen, that we MUST DEFEAT the motion; You are only HURTING yourself; You are only hurting YOURSELF; I WOULDN'T DO that if I were you; I wouldn't DO that if I were YOU.

phasizing other words. You can also work on this list for practice."[2]

[2] *FOR-ward, MARCH; To BE or NOT to be, THAT is the QUES-tion; FOR the people, BY the people, OF the people; It's TOO EARLY to leave NOW; It took TWENTY HOURS to get home from Chicago; Driving in the RAIN is NO FUN; I had a REAL GOOD TIME at your party; He's ALWAYS on TOP of the job; a WORD to the WISE; as GOOD as GOLD; Look AROUND all you WISH.*

Make up sentences that refer to the business or special interest of the patient.

Final Instructions to the Patient

"We have reached the end of our formal instructions on esophageal speech. This does not mean that you may drop all practice and forget the many points that we have given you. It is important to keep improving your speech for several years. If you don't talk much, or practice, you won't improve. We know of persons who recorded their speech once a year for five years. Their speech improved over each preceding year. Another point to remember is to keep all appointments with your surgeon, and never miss a checkup. This is important for your health and your emotional security. Finally, we urge you to continue to come to our Lost Chord Club meetings. You will serve as an example of recovery from cancer, and will be an inspiration to other patients who will come in the future. There are many things that you can do for others at the club. You will always be able to 'Thank God that He gave you two voices in a single lifetime.' "

To the speech clinician: At this point, give periodic Test 7 (page 98).

GROUP THERAPY FOR TEACHING ESOPHAGEAL SPEECH

Many Lost Chord Clubs evolved from a cluster of patients whom one devoted teacher had taught and later brought together for inspiration and group practice. The same situation occurs today whenever a strong, successful esophageal speaker finds a number of fellow laryngectomees who live within a reasonable driving distance from a common center. Thus, from the beginning, many instructors of groups of laryngectomees have been laryngectomized persons. About one-half of the clubs today have laryngectomized instructors exclusively. One-quarter of them have speech pathologists and the remainder have both types of instructors serving them.

Group therapy for postlaryngectomy speech may consist of formal instruction of two or more persons, or a less formal instruction of a larger group. The class might be the assembled members of a Lost Chord Club, or the patients in a speech and hearing center which uses only group instruction. When only two or three are instructed as a group, the instructor has more time and opportunity to pay closer attention to the development of each member's speech. When the group consists of a large number of patients, the instructor cannot handle specific speech problems in detail unless he selects certain cases with whom he can point out faulty speech and demonstrate special techniques for correction, which all of the group can then work out for themselves. It is thus possible for some members to learn to talk as quickly as they would with individual practice, provided that they practice what they observe.*

Although all of the techniques in this text are available for group sessions, it is wiser for the instructor to begin simple relaxation and breathing exercises. An audience-participation exercise may be used to demonstrate normal tonicity in muscles, as contrasted with muscle tension. For example, members may be divided into pairs, one of whom is requested to rest his hand on the outstretched index finger of his partner. When the instructor says, "Now!" the partner quickly withdraws his finger. The other member observes that he keeps his hand and arm extended as if they were still supported. Next, the instructor tells the first member to let his hand and arm go limp until he feels that only the index finger is holding the arm up. When the finger is withdrawn this time, the hand will fall more promptly. Next, the instructor requests everyone to clasp their hands together and grip them very hard, and suddenly relax them. Finally, he asks everyone to tighten and screw up the face muscles and squint the eyes tightly for a moment and then let them go. He then explains that the first part of each exercise demonstrated how people tighten up with fear and tensions, and that the second part demonstrated that muscles felt much looser when they were relaxed. The latter way is how they should be when laryngectomees are talking.

Another action is to instruct the members to inhale and nod the head backward, and then sigh as they drop the head forward. The head should definitely drop as if no muscles hold it up. Another procedure to get the

---

*We believe that anyone who uses the group to save time and money will do a disservice to the patients. A time comes when every patient needs individual attention and encouragement.

class in a relaxed mood is to ask everyone to laugh. They are puzzled over this request because they think they cannot laugh. Then have everyone say *ah-ah-ah*. This is equivalent to *hah-hah-hah*. If laryngectomees can train themselves to do this when a joke is heard, they will make sounds of laughter instead of just blowing from the stomas. Members will be asked to tell a joke, after which everyone is requested to laugh vocally.

The instructor may have the members prolong different vowels, consonant-vowel syllables and the many combinations that are found in the manuals on teaching alaryngeal speech. (See the Appendix for manuals that are available). Each member may be requested to say several vowels or syllables. Competition may be set up to determine how many can get air in and out in an acceptable length of time. New members and slow speakers will be inspired to produce sounds faster after they see that others are doing it. Practice in groups and then in competition will prove that there are marked differences. Competition makes the class interesting to the older members. Counting the largest number of digits is another feat for competition. If the instructor records the rates on the blackboard, he as well as the class, will, observe a cluster around a certain figure. Each member will see where he stands in the group.

Articulation of all consonants, as well as of vowels, in words, phrases and syllables will improve accuracy. An effective stunt is to have everyone count from 21 to 30. The instructor exaggerates, in fact overexaggerates, with his lips to stimulate the members to articulate more accurately. First, they whisper while exaggerating with their lips, then they count aloud. The whisper is not forced; rather it is designed to develop awareness of labial and lingual action. Members are next requested to count aloud, using the exaggerated action. They are urged to practice this every morning, counting up to 100. This increases their intelligibility and gives the impression that they are talking louder.

The speech clinician can make the sessions more productive and interesting by giving the physiological basis of each sound with which patients have difficulty. For example, he may state that the voice of one of the members tends to fade out at the end of a word, that is, he does not voice a final sound, such as the final sound of *judge*. He then demonstrates that the tongue should be held against the upper front teeth until the consonant is completely voiced. Also, the members are requested to indicate if they hear the other members' final consonants. (Keep in mind that some may be hard of hearing.)

Many techniques that are used in individual instruction may be used, though of course not all at one session. Accent, emphasis, prolonging phrases, improving fluency, vowel accuracy, etc., may be rewarding activities. Indeed, they can become dramatic. Singing is excellent, especially if a pianist is available, but good work can be done without one. An effective demonstration to observers is to have the class first read a stanza of a song in unison, sing it and again read it aloud. The last reading usually appears to have much more naturalness in rhythm and continuity, as well as being more intelligible.

Another competition is to test the reading rate of the members by giving them a simple passage of about 150 words. Every tenth word is numbered above the line. The members are started reading on signal, in unison, but at their own rates. It may seem like bedlam but it has a purpose. They are told to stop reading after one minute, then they are requested to count the number of words read. The instructor records the results on a scale. He informs them that sixty words per minute is acceptable for training class graduates but that it will reach one hundred and more with practice. Snidecor states that a rate of 125 words per minute is the average for good speakers. The results may be an added stimulus to reach higher goals. It is advisable to retain these results for later comparisons.

Stunts, imitations of great orators and displays of great emotion can be introduced. The instructor may write one word on the board and ask someone to use it in a sentence to demonstrate emotion. For example, the word *sick* may be demonstrated by the expression, "You make me sick," or "I am sorry you are sick." Other words such as *cold, full, well, sorry, angry,* etc., may be used. Someone may be asked to conduct an auction of some white elephants or humorous items. Motions can be made, seconded and argued vociferously. Members can wave their hands, stand up and talk back during an argument, all in fun. Different members may take turns reading the club prayer. Such participation is designed to encourage all members to express themselves more freely with the hope that they will engage in more oral activity at home. Most important is the development of everyone's willingness to talk. Since tension arises under conditions of excitement, the speakers may learn to reduce this in their oral activities at the group sessions.

SUPPLEMENTARY TECHNIQUES FOR TEACHING ESOPHAGEAL SPEECH

No two successive patients can be treated exactly alike by a speech clinician, because their problems are never identical. Their personalities are different and they may respond to the same instructions in a different manner. It is quite appropriate, therefore, that we present some techniques that have been found to be successful with some patients when other techniques were not. These are by no means all of the techniques that are available. Speech clinicians may have some of their own which have not been made public. All of these techniques may be potentially advantageous to one patient or another.

Unit 37. Encouraging the Patient

By the time you have met the patient several times at the hospital, pre- or postoperatively, and have started his lessons, you should know his stability, whether he is discouraged and wants to quit or is anxious to go on. You must know whether he is working on his speech; his spouse should be able to tell you. If he is discouraged, praise him on each little success. Never lose your enthusiasm. Likewise, urge him and his wife to go to the Lost Chord Club meetings, and emphasize that even though he is not talking, he should go to observe others.

If the patient is living alone, explain to him the importance of being with people daily, at the store, at meetings, with relatives or friends. If he does nothing else, he should practice his exercises out loud hundreds of times. Later, he should be encouraged to read out loud daily. An interesting self-entertainment which is a profitable effort is imitating the speech of people who talk on television or radio programs. Even imitating the emotions of these people is profitable self-education. If tape recordings or disc recordings are available (Doehler; Hyman), the speech clinician should use them to demonstrate what other laryngectomees have achieved. Shanks (1967) recommends making periodic recordings of the patients to demonstrate gains in accuracy and fluency.

Unit 38. The Whistle Technique

To the speech clinician: A patient can be trained to become aware of movement of air backward into the pharynx and perhaps into the neoglottis by blowing a toy whistle (from a cereal package) with a very small opening (1 x 8 mm) that permits him to build up air pressure for the production of an esophageal sound (Gardner 1962a).[1] When the patient tries to force air forward against the small opening, some of it will move backward into the pharynx and esophagus. This may be similar to the phenomenon of the movement into the esophagus of some of the air made during the production of /s/ (Diedrich and Youngstrom).[2]

[1] Caution: A whistle with a large opening will not work. The idea is to produce enough air pressure in the mouth to cause some of it to be moved backward.

[2] It would be helpful to read Diedrich and Youngstrom on the phenomenon of air splitting during the production of /s/. Also see the presentation of /s/ in Unit 10.

"Here is a tiny whistle with a very small opening. It requires a great deal of pressure to make a loud, sharp sound. I drop my tongue tip down as if to make a /t/ sound. This action forces the air against the whistle opening. Not all of the air can get through; some of it moves back into my throat. If I relax my throat as I blow, I feel the air going into my esophagus. It may be possible for you to relax in the same way to let the air in. We first will help you to feel the backward movement of air.

"Watch me. I'll blow the whistle. I must get a sharp whistle. You try your whistle. ... Close the lips tightly around it. Put your tongue against your upper front teeth as if to say /t/. As your tongue compresses air, drop it sharply forward to force air into the whistle.[3] Try it. ... You blew air from the stoma. All of the work is done inside your mouth with the tongue and the whistle. Try it once more. ... You got a tiny whistle. Try it again. Concentrate the air at that tiny opening and force it through! Be sure to open up your throat at the moment you whistle. Try it again. ... Drop the back of the tongue as you do in a yawn, while the tongue makes the whistle. That really makes me yawn. ... Good. You got a whistle.[4] Again, think what you are supposed to do. You must compress air and move some of it back. Instead of using only the tongue, you can use the whistle to move the air back. Let's do the sharp whistle five times. ... Good. You are coming along nicely. Did you feel the air move into your throat? ... Then do this next. After you whistle and feel the air moving down, immediately bring back that air to say *ah*. Whistle, say *ah*. ... Once more. ... Again. ... and again. ...

"Another way of doing the sound after the compression is to blow air out as you whisper *woot* or *whoot*.[5] As you blow air, you say *whoot* and relax the throat. Whoosh the air through the tiny hole of the rounded lips.[6] ...

[3] Some patients are able to blow with the tongue flat and feel the air enter the throat.

[4] Some patients may have to practice in an adjoining room or take the whistle home for practice.

[5] Some patients have formed their own nonsense syllable for producing the forward flow of air and the backward flow of part of it. They may say *whoot* as they open the throat.

[6] Analysis of this action indicates that it is the tongue action for injecting. So if the patient says *whoot* and completes injection, he should recognize the pattern.

You whisper the sound, you don't say the vowel aloud. Try it. ... Try *whip,* leaving out the vowel, but making a sharp closing action of the lips as the voiceless consonants are whipped out and the throat is opened. ... This time, simply protrude your lips, then compress them together, which forces out the air. Most of it goes backward. ... Good, you have several new methods, all working toward compression. Take the whistle home with you [or to an adjoining room] and practice until you get a good action.

"The next action is to get the air back up. Blow the whistle and say *ah.*[7] ... Say the voiceless *whoot,*[8] feeling the air go down, and then say *ah.* ... Practice all of these and I'll see you after a while. This time we will not move the air through the lips, but will go through the motions. We compress the air around the rounded lips and force it backward into the pharynx. All of the air goes back; none goes out. Let's clinch the action by compressing the air with the lips and cheeks and saying *tah.* ... Again. ... Now we are getting the correct method of injecting air, aided by explosive action."

[7] Of course, the whistle is quickly withdrawn after blowing so that the mouth is opened for *ah.*

[8] It is obvious that you should work on these suggested sounds so that you can express your own experience to the patient. You may find other sound combinations that work better.

Unit 39. Opening an Overly Tense PE Segment

True esophageal sound can be produced only by injecting air into and expelling air out of the esophagus. If the mouth of the esophagus does not open, injection and expulsion cannot occur. Tonic closure of the mouth of the cricopharyngeal sphincter (neoglottis) is a natural reflex action which normally prevents inhaled air from entering the esophagus of a person who has his larynx. The efforts of a laryngectomee to talk by whispering forcefully may occasionally force closure of the neoglottis. Damsté; Diedrich and Youngstrom; M.C.L. Greene, and others reported that even the effort to use plosive consonants may cause this undesirable closure in some patients. This condition may also be the reason why some patients use pharyngeal speech. Damsté recommends that if it is suspected that a neoglottic spasm is present, the speech clinician should refrain from further effort to obtain esophageal speech until the PE segment can be opened by one or more of the following measures:

1. Relaxation of neck, shoulder and facial muscles (Damsté; M.C.L. Greene).

2. Broad yawning, quick inhalation and sudden thrusting of the jaw forward to open the neoglottis (Damsté; Gatewood; Luchsinger and Arnold; Moore). Repeated phonation should follow the successful opening of the esophagus to fixate the action and build kinesthetic imagery.

3. Forcing air into the esophagus by pressing a bulb. A catheter is inserted through the nose and thence into the neoglottis. The patient is requested to say *ah* as soon as he feels the air enter the esophagus; in order to establish a reflex action. After the catheter is removed, the patient repeatedly injects air and says *ah* (Berlin 1963a; Damsté; Gatewood; M.C.L. Greene; Luchsinger and Arnold; Seeman 1967; Snidecor). The technique is regarded as giving psychological encouragement to the patient who has not been successful with injection. It also gives the patient a kinesthetic image of the pressure in the esophagus which he must feel prior to injection (Gatewood).

4. Catheter dilation of the esophagus by having the patient swallow a weighted catheter of a given size. Larger and larger catheters are inserted from time to time until the laryngologist decides that the neoglottis can function (Arnold; Damsté; Damsté *et al.*; Gatewood; Luchsinger and Arnold). Therapy can then be resumed in a manner that will not re-create tension in the throat.

5. Having the patient breathe out all air, cover the stoma with a bunched handkerchief, then inspire quickly and yawn broadly simultaneously, after which he says *ah*. The patient should be asked to feel the entrance of the air. He may be told to "suck" the air into the throat.

6. Using warm drinks, coarse food, chewing gum and hard candy to develop enough stretching and/or relaxing of the esophagus to permit it to open (Harrington; Snidecor).

As a preliminary precaution, Diedrich and Youngstrom suggest that the speech clinician find out if the patient is truly practicing his speech program. It is occasionally discovered that the patient is not working on the lessons at home.

Unit 40. Eliminating Repetitive Movements of the Lips, Jaw and Head on Air Intake

Unnecessary or repetitive movements of the lips and jaw, and nodding of the head during the effort to inject air, are signals that the patient is having difficulty in taking in air, or that he is not sure he has taken in enough air for the impending production. This action is most apparent when the patient is requested to say a longer word or more syllables than he thinks he can say in one air-charge. The following steps should be helpful in overcoming these problems:

1. Explaining the causes of this behavior. The speech clinician should ask the patient why he makes the repetitive movements. The patient often cannot explain why, because he does not know he is making them. When he observes himself in a mirror, he is surprised. He then may admit that he is unsure of himself.

2. Checking on coordination of respiration and phonation (M.C.L. Greene).

3. Using the sniff technique for obtaining greater air intake (Diedrich and Youngstrom).

4. Prolonging the vowels in syllables that begin with plosive consonants, e.g., *pie,* and alternating with syllables that have no plosive consonants, e.g., *my.*

5. Teaching the patient to move his lips and tongue more rapidly so that he can make more sounds in a given time. First use diphthongs. The patient will be surprised that he can glide from vowel to vowel in one air-charge. Follow the first steps by increasing the number of syllables that can be spoken in a given time. Confidence is thus increased; the patient will not be nervous and will not begin to bob his head again.

6. Instructing the patient to relax on the first syllables in a word so that he will have enough air left for the last part of the word or phrase.

Unit 41. Correction of Grimaces, Tensions and Strains

Numerous voice patients have admitted that they do well at home but that as soon as they enter the clinic they begin to tighten up because they are anxious to make a good showing for their teacher. We have found this to be especially true of our dysphonic patients. Lifting the eyebrows, twitching the lips and blinking the eyelids indicate that the patient is trying too hard; his tension is spreading from the speech muscles to the neck muscles. His general tension as indicated by grimaces may also spread to his neck muscles, which interferes with the normal function of the speech mechanism. Likewise, he may be too anxious or insecure, or he may not understand what he is supposed to do. Relaxation exercises are useful for the laryngectomee. The speech clinician may talk quietly to the patient and explain why tension prevents him from doing well. After he is more at ease, instruction should be resumed.

Coordination of diaphragmatic breathing with an easy relaxed phonation should be developed. At first, the patient must be trained to say *ah* as lightly as he can, that is, not forcefully. (This does not refer to audibility.) Inhalation before injection generally reduces the chance of tension interrupting the phonation, especially if the patient has learned to breathe out slowly as though he is sighing. We have seen extra movements diminish when the patient sees himself in a mirror. Much of the tension centers around the climactic moment of saying the esophageal sound. This is quite apparent when the patient hesitates, rolls his eyes, searches for some saliva or looks around before he injects or makes the sound. This is why some laryngectomees keep a lozenge in their mouth at all times.

Diedrich and Youngstrom have recommended the use of body movements to initiate the esophageal sound. They suggest that the patient should walk while he is making the effort. He should imitate an underhand pitch of a ball at the moment he initiates the sound. We have found these movements very helpful with beginning speakers and with patients who have fixated certain bad habits.* Household tasks such as swinging a broom or pushing an iron, might be tied in with the initial effort. Froeschels' pushing exercises may also be tried. Later, these accessory activities must be diminished to the point where they are merely imaginary, until eventually the patient is free of the bad habits. We cannot emphasize too much that the patient must understand that the speech sounds are made inside the mouth and that the external movements of eyebrows and eyelids have nothing to do with effecting production of esophageal sounds.

Unit 42. Eliminating Stoma Noise

Some patients have great difficulty in eliminating the natural reflex of breathing out rapidly during speech. This should be handled in the early stages of therapy by emphasizing that the speech activity is inside the mouth and throat and has no direct relation to breathing out. The methods listed below may be used to correct the habit:

1. When a hearing loss is present, the patient should be provided with feedback (a TOK-BAK device, stethoscope, amplifier with receivers, etc.). When he hears how loudly he blows, he will quickly learn to reduce the stoma noise.

2. Another striking method is holding one end of a rubber tube over the stoma and the other end near the speaker's face, eye or ear. When he blows he will feel the forceful expiration and quickly reduce the flow.

3. The patient should be made to inhale and sigh slowly, then

---

*These patterns remind us of the distraction releases of the stutterer. Here, they appear to be reinforcement patterns.

inject air and sigh slowly as he says *pah*. Next he should repeat monosyllables as he slowly sighs.

4. The patient should be requested to count by continuous lip whispering as he breathes in and out slowly. He should be cautioned against heavy, forced breathing or a breathy whisper. He may also raise his hand on inspiration and lower it slowly during expiration. Then he should start to count with voice while he is slowly lowering his hand; this will tend to slow his exhalation.

5. An occasional patient will blow air loudly from his stoma as a result of trying to utilize that last bit of air in his lungs to complete a word or sentence. He should be requested to observe what he does as he repeats the sentence in question. It should be made clear to him that it is better to take in air more frequently and finish his words than to end the word or sentence in silence, or with a wheeze from the stoma. Practicing with one easy injection per syllable, followed by two and eventually more syllables, will demonstrate what is wanted. Counting and increasing the numbers per air-charge is helpful.

Unit 43. Correction for Substitution of Sounds

Speech clinicians report that laryngectomees substitute voiced for voiceless sounds and vice versa under varying conditions (Diedrich and Youngstrom; Shames *et al.*; Snidecor; Tikofsky *et al.*). Since /k/ is spoken more easily at the end of a word (Diedrich and Youngstrom), the patient should work with one-syllable words that have voiced and unvoiced endings, such as *beck-beg, back-bag, tuck-tug* and *luck-lug*, in order to develop the kinesthetic and auditory differences of the two final sounds. The discrimination may be learned more quickly by using an auditory training unit with which the patient hears first the teacher's voice and then his own. A hearing aid will also serve the same purpose.

To improve the production of initial /k/, the sound may be repeated two or more times before the word is finally pronounced, e.g., *k-k-kit*. A syllable or word that ends in /k/ may be given the first time, followed by a syllable that begins with /k/, e.g., *take-cake*. At the end of the word, the patient may repeat the /k/ or /g/ two or three times, e.g., *keg-g-g* or *kick-k-k*. The patient should exaggerate the /k/ and /g/ sounds and should be sure that he hears the differences. Likewise, the clinician may use a syllable ending in a /g/ to precede one beginning with /k/, as in *egg-keg*. In all situations, the clinician should be sure that the initial /k/ is clearly pronounced in spite of its blending with the following vowel (Snidecor).

Lists of words should be prepared to contrast the endings of voiceless and voiced sounds. Some examples are *tag-tack, bid-bit, tab-tap* and *save-safe*. The speech clinician may wish to improve discrimination between these sounds in the same way he did with the /k/ sounds.

Unit 44. Correcting Excessive Air Intake

Patients who take in an excessive quantity of air complain of great discomfort (bloating of air in the stomach) and tend to make explosive sounds from the esophagus (Martin 1963). (A very tight or tense esophagus may also contribute to explosive action and poor articulation.) This condition is common among patients who have been taught to swallow. When these patients understand what is happening, they are usually willing to work with plosive-laden syllables, which help to eliminate the need for heavy swallowing and to reduce the amount of air intake necessary to produce the desired esophageal sound.

In our clinical experience, we have helped patients reduce excessive air intake by using plosives in the initial and medial positions. The patient is taught to make the injection quickly and to produce the esophageal sounds as fast as possible. We emphasize the in-fast, out-fast technique (Snidecor) and explain that the dual action is actually a complete cycle of continuous action. The speech clinician may also take advantage of the air intake (not the air in the stomach) to train the patient to double or treble the number of syllables that he can say in one air intake. (This is possible if the esophagus is large and properly controlled.)

Unit 45. Eliminating Noisy Air Intake

A klunking sound,* accompanying air intake, is often heard in beginning esophageal speakers. The patient may be hard of hearing and may not hear himself making the sound. A stethoscope placed near the area of the esophagus, with the earpiece inserted in the ear of the patient, will let him hear the klunking. The clinician should demonstrate an easy air intake and explain that the patient need not try so hard. Repetition of *pah* or other plosive-laden syllables can prove to him that it is not necessary to inject so forcefully. The patient should sniff lightly and make an easy injection before each number as he counts from 1 to 10. He then should increase the number of figures he can say with one air intake that is not noisy. The clinician should talk to him in an easy, relaxed manner, explaining that tension causes many voice problems, then have him inhale easily and sigh several times, reminding him to relax. The patient should then inhale and inject easily. This is very helpful in establishing a much easier and less noisy intake of air. Finally, if he continues to have a noisy

---

*The word klinkers is used by the speech class at the University of Kansas Medical Center (Diedrich and Youngstrom).

air intake, he may have to replace injection with inhalation. In fact, the effort to inhale may be sufficient to break down the habit of klunking.

Unit 46. Eliminating the Pharyngeal Voice

It should be unnecessary to discuss the pharyngeal voice as a type, because it is rarely observed. Some writers (Damsté; Diedrich and Youngstrom; Gardner; M.C.L. Greene; Hodson and Oswald) have heard at least one pharyngeal voice. However, students may read about this in the early literature, where some writers in reality were describing esophageal voice. (See our discussion on types of laryngeal speech.) Another reason is that some patients may first appear to use pharyngeal speech during the process of trying to learn esophageal speech. This later changes to true esophageal speech. This has occurred at some of the IAL voice institutes. Damsté has also mentioned this possibility. Hence, the speech clinician should be forewarned about the specific nature of this type of voice.

The basic problem of the speaker may be a very tight closure of the PE segment, or excessive scar formation which may prevent the speaker from injecting air into the esophagus (Luchsinger and Arnold). In other words, he has no esophageal air to produce voice. Hence, he develops a substitute location for making the vibration, namely, between the tongue and the wall of the pharynx or between other parts such as the soft palate and tonsil pillars. The hypopharynx may then serve as the air chamber.

Damsté *et al.* described the high-pitched, squeaking, weak voice that was created in the pharyngeal area. The patient was unable to make the initial vowel, and could not make a belch. Frequent short interruptions of sound were needed to reload the pseudoglottis. Since the tongue had the task of creating the sound, it was impossible for the sound to be modified in the usual resonant chambers. If it is possible to alter the pharyngeal voice, it may be called a temporary pharyngeal voice. If therapy cannot change the voice, it should be regarded as pathological (Damsté).

The first goal for correction is to obtain an esophageal sound; that is, the patient must get air into the esophagus. He may try a true swallow, usually with water or a carbonated drink, to get the feeling of air going deeper into the throat and to get air back up, in contrast to the squeezing effect between the tongue and opposing surfaces. The speech clinician may also assume that the patient has not yet learned esophageal voice, and may proceed to develop it in the usual manner.

The speech clinician may use inhalation, especially a strong sniff through the nose, simultaneously with inhalation directly into the stoma and mouth. The air is drawn into the esophagus so that words, preferably containing plosives, may be said simultaneously with expulsion. Damsté used plosive-laden words that had the accent on the second, syllable, such as *cartoon, pertain* and *pontoon.* In his difficult cases, he obtained esophageal speech only after dilating the esophagus and training the patient to release the air gradually and consciously.

Unit 47. Speech Problems of the Patient with Excessive Loss of Tissue

The most outstanding types of laryngectomy where excessive tissue has been removed are pharyngolaryngectomy and esophagectomy. In the former type, the cancer involves both the pharyngeal area and the larynx. In the latter it involves the upper one-third of the esophagus and the larynx (Luchsinger and Arnold). In the case of esophagectomy, the upper one-third of the esophagus and the larynx are removed. Plastic surgery, spread over many weeks, is designed to build a new esophagus and to attach it to the caudal end of the hypopharynx. However, the PE sphincter is missing; hence, there is little possibility of obtaining neurological or physiological control of the esophagus to serve as an air chamber from which air is expelled. Under such circumstances, the clinician must resort to trial and error to devise some means of developing air compression and injection. The most common technique is to use digital pressure on the area of the PE junction to narrow the tube enough to obtain minimal vibration. Wearing a small bit of sponge rubber against that area may help. It may be held in place by a tape that is tied behind the neck. Inflation at best is very small. We have had several patients who were able to produce a semblance of an esophageal sound, but it would be absurd to say that we had succeeded in obtaining serviceable speech. Inhalation is probably the best method of air intake for these people.

M.C.L. Greene reports that one of her patients talked on both air intake and expulsion. The resulting voice was quite breathy and husky, and had very little vibratory quality. Our philosophy on this type of voice problem is that it is an injustice to the patient to deprive him of the early communication he can get by using an artificial larynx, especially since he has to endure frequent surgical revisions that may extend from six months to a year or more. We have known patients who were persuaded to persist in efforts to develop air-charge and oral expression for two years, during which no suggestion was made that they could communicate with an artificial larynx. We have obtained some phonation from several patients of this type, but never enough to produce more than one syllable per air-charge. The vocal product was barely audible, and several seconds elapsed between each sound unit.

If pharyngeal or glossal tissue is removed, the problem is still more complicated. The only procedure that the speech clinician can use is to resort to all the methods of voice, resonance and articulation known to the profession, in addition to the therapy usually used for laryngectomees. Again, we suggest that the patient be given an opportunity to communicate by means of an artificial larynx, and that he be trained to use his residual articulators with as much skill as he can generate. He thus can communicate during the period in which he is endeavoring to develop an esophageal type of speech. Finally, use of the instrument may enable the patient to develop good action for voiceless consonants; he can utilize these new patterns for any esophageal speech he may eventually develop after months of persistent effort.

your thumb ready to press the knob. Now, say *ah* as you press the knob. ... Good. That sounded like *ah*, didn't it? ... Let's move the disc around to other spots.[5] Say *ah* each time as you press the knob. ... Right there gives a good sound. Learn to keep it on that spot for the present."

Unit 49. Using Voiced Sounds: Vowels

"Vowels are easy to say. Exaggerate with your lips and jaw to say them.[1] Keep the mouth open wider than usual so that the sound comes out. There is no breath stream to project it forward. Press the knob and say /a/ (*ah*). ... Good. Hold the vowel longer one time, release the knob, then hold it shorter, release the knob, then again hold it longer, like this: *aaaaaaaaaaah*. ... *aaaaah*. ... *aaaaaaaaaaaah*. ... That was good. Here's another vowel: /u/ (*oo*). Say *ooooooo*, holding that the same way. ... Let's say five long vowels like this: *may*. ... *me*. ... *my*. ... *moh*. ... *moo*. ... Be sure to press to start sound and release the moment you are through. Do those vowel-words over. Shape your lips so that I can see what vowel you are saying. Start with *may* again. ... That's fine. Practice on the vowels at home.

"We have some double vowels; we call them dipthongs. You say two vowels quickly, blending them as one. All you need to do is shape the two sounds quickly with your lips and tongue and the vibrator will do the rest of the phonation. Here is one: /au/ (*ow*). Do it like this: *ah-oo*. ... Good. Now prolong each sound and quickly glide from one to the other. ... Here's another dipthong, /aɪ/ (*i*) as in *ride*. You glide from *ah* to *ee*,[2] *aaaaaaaaaaaaeeeeeeeee*. Try it. ... Hold the knob down as long as you vibrate; it is not a matter of breathing. Do that dipthong five times, pausing after each one. ... Now, say five of them rapidly without pausing; you keep the vibrator down all through them. ... That shows you can talk rapidly while the

[5] The sound may be quite different, weaker or stronger at different spots.

[1] Start with vowels because the sound is already available through the instrument, and you can show the patient that he can talk at once. Shaping the lips for the vowels increases the activity of the articulators and at the same time gives the patient a feeling that he is having less difficulty talking than he thought he would.

[2] Although research may show that speech with an artificial larynx may be more intelligible than esophageal speech, this does not mean that the speaker has complete intelligibility with the instrument. Hence, it is necessary to work with both vowels and consonants with the artificial larynx (Diedrich and Youngstrom).

knob is down. Try this one: /ɔi/ (*aw-ee*). Say it like this: awawawawaweeeeee. ... Now say the two, blended together, rapidly, five of them without pause. ... Be sure to shape the lips carefully.

"Let's put /m/ before the vowel, as in *ma*. Firm your lips for /m/ and press the knob. ... You got a good sound. Start with /m/ and hold *ma* longer. ... Now say *mama*. ... Prolong that one to *maaaaamaaaa*. ... Try *moo-moo*. ... *may-may*. ... *my-my*. ... *mee-mee*. ... Put the /m/ on the end of the syllable and be sure to keep the knob pressed down until after you finish the /m/ *mahm*. ... *maim*. ... *mome*. ... *home*. ... You hesitated on /h/ in *home*. That is not really pronounced, but you shape your lips for the vowel. Say *home* again and hold the vibrator a little longer to get feeling for final /m/. ... That's good.

"Let's do the same with /n/. Say *now*. ... *noo*. ... *nine*. ... *noon*. ... *noun*. ... *moon*. ... *name*. ... *man*. ... *moon-man*. ... Good.[3]

"Before you go, tell me how you have been communicating with your family and friends. ... Do you realize it is no longer necessary for you to write on a pad? ... Start talking all you wish to with this instrument. But if you do write something, keep the notes and show them to me."

Unit 50. Breathing and Stoma Noise

"Let's have the notes you wrote out since I last saw you. ... Some of these are words that you could have said with the instrument. You wrote: *Are you taking the car?* Let's say that with the instrument.[1] ... No problem at all. Here's another: *Has the mail come?* Try that. ... No problem. And you wrote out, *What's the matter with Tommy?* Try that. ... You are not making the consonants as clear as they should be but you are communicating and that is important.[2] I urge you to telephone friends and

[3] Practice words for vowels:

him; home; noun; harm; none; bone; omen; man; me; my; may; men; moon; mule; name; mail; maim; dame; dime; down; mamma; Mamie; Hey- man; no man; new man; my man; mamma's man; moon man; my name; new name; aim now; own home; new noun; no noun; home no more.

[1] You should say the sentences first.

[2] This also helps the patient get back on the job sooner than if he waited until he could talk again.

relatives. It is no problem. You hold your mouth near the mouthpiece just as before. The sound comes out there. Be sure to identify yourself when the person answers the phone. He will be more attentive that way and won't mistake you for someone else.

"You are making a lot of noise from your stoma when you talk. It is a natural reaction because your lungs sent up the air through the larynx, throat and mouth to give you voice. Blowing won't help you now. Put your instrument on the desk. We will first inhale and sigh slowly. ... Rest the palms of your hands on the lower ribs and your fingers over that soft spot just below your breast bone. That triangular area is called the substernal or epigastric area.[3] Now breathe in and feel your abdomen moving out and pushing your hands. When you breathe out, as in speaking, it moves inward. Putting your hands there helps you to become aware of what you do when you breathe during speech, if you breathe correctly. Inhale at the beginning of a sentence and between phrases, just as you did in normal speech. When you speak with the instrument, you can't use lung air but you can breathe out slowly. Then you won't blow loudly. Do this: Inhale quickly and then count mentally to 5 as you slowly breathe out.[4] Feel the abdomen moving slowly back in. ... To learn how to do it while using the instrument, inhale and count slowly with it from 1 to 5. Do that three times. ... Good. Now, let's hear you count up to 10 while breathing out slowly. ... That's better. Watch your breathing and if you hear yourself blowing, know that it is not necessary. You can't use lung air to talk with an instrument.

"Let's go back to saying vowels. Say *ma-ma-ma-ma*. Do it ten times, slowly breathing out. ... What happened to that soft triangle? Forgot to watch it? And you lifted your shoulders instead. Let's watch it this time. Take in

[3] Some help will be given to the patient by demonstrating the technique for him. It is important that he be aware of the abdomen moving slowly inward as he talks. An effective demonstration is to hold the end of a book against the abdomen and have the patient watch it move in as he talks and breathes out slowly.

[4] Another method is to have the patient count aloud as he slowly raises his hand. This, associated with slow breathing, enables him to dissociate the blowing from speech.

a quick sniff and sigh out slowly as you count to ten. ... That's the way your air should move out, and you didn't blow. Well, let's try again with *ma-ma-ma-ma-ma*. Remember to speak the five words at your natural pace while slowly moving out the air. Try it. ... That's much better. Remember how you do it.[5] When you are talking with people, regulate the slow breathing even though you are talking rapidly."

[5] Some users of the artificial larynx are able to talk continuously by completely dissociating their breathing from their speech. They may not even pause for logical expression, but waggle their tongues without cessation.

Unit 51. Using Voiced Consonants: /w/, /l/ and /r/

"Today we are going to work on voiced consonants. Your lips and tongue will shape the vibrated sound into whatever consonants you desire to make. We will start with /w/, /l/ and /r/. For /w/, you start the vibrator as you round your lips and quickly glide to the following vowel. The glide consists of dropping the jaw quickly, a lot or a little depending on the vowel. Say /uwʌ/ (*oowuh*). ... Now say just /wʌ/ (*wuh*). ... Say /uwi/ (*oo-wee*). ... Then /wi/ (*wee*). ... Now say *way-wee-wye-woe-woo*. ... Make up a list of words that have the sound /w/ in the middle (e.g., *sidewalk, highway*) to add to this list of words.[1]

"In order to make /l/ correctly with the instrument, you must hold the tip of the tongue against the back of the upper teeth throughout the vibration of the instrument. Let's try it that way. Put the tongue up there, start the vibrator and hold the tongue until the vibrator stops. ... This time, say *lah-lah-lah-lah-lah* and keep the vibrator down throughout. ... Do it again but stop the vibrator after each syllable. ... In the word *Hello*, prolong the /l/ by keeping the vibrator going and then glide to the *oh*. ... Say it once more: *Hellllo*. ... Now, say *holy* the same way. ... *jolllly*. ... *Polllly*. ... Say *lay-lee-lye-low-loo* with continuous vibration. ... Take this list of words and emphasize the /l/.[2]

"It's helpful to start making the /r/ sound

[1] *way; wee; wye; woe; woo; win; wit; wine; women; won; wane; wean; wen; away; awoke; always; bow wow; anyway; highway; anyone; someone; Wee Winnie won one.*

Count from 1 to 20, then from 20 to 29.

[2] *lane; line; lamb; lump; lap; lip; all; ale; ill; mill; limb; mill; hill; hole; holy; hello; holly; Millie; Mollie; Tillie; lean; kneel; Nellie; lily; lolly; lonely; homely; lime; limen; lemon.*

first by saying *ah* and gliding to the /r/ by curling the tongue tip slightly. Do it this way: Start the vibrator as you say *ah* and hold it two seconds, then curl the tongue up for /r/. It sounds like *ah-ir*. Then prolong the vibrator for the /r/. Say *ah-irr*. ... Good. Say *ah-ir-run*. ... *ah-ir-roar*. ... *ah-ir-rear*. ... Now, say *run-roar-rear* with continuous vibration. ... If you hold your tongue correctly, the vibrator does the work. Let's pay attention to /r/ at the end of the word. Keep the vibrator going through the /r/ in *fear*. ... *near*. ... *tear*. ... Work on this list of words to get a definite feeling of how /r/ is made with the tongue curled up and the vibrator going."[3]

[3] *roar; rare; rear; roam; run; roan; lear; real; roll; near; nor; norm; normal; hurry; Harry; Larry; holler; rumor; roamer; room; rummer; roller; harelip; collar; caller; color; dollar; paper boy; prayer room; pain reliever; rubber mat; proper manner; pepper pot; triphammer; paper trimmer; paper carrier; newspaper.*

Unit 52. Introducing Voiced and Voiceless Plosives

"Tell me how much note writing you've done lately. ... None? That's good news. Then you can talk to anyone any time. Have you used the telephone? ... Well, why don't you try it? Have you had any people misunderstanding you? ... Then you might expect that to happen over the telephone. Let's get some practice right now. Cup your hand as if it were the receiver. You have dialed the number; when someone answers, ask for the fare and time schedule to Milwaukee. ... That went off nicely. From now on, don't hesitate to call friends and relatives. You will be understood.

"Let's work on /b/, /d/ and /g/ sounds. Say *bay*. ... *bee*. ... *buy*. ... *boe*. ... *booo*. ... *day-dee-die*. ... *doe-due daw*. ... Try these: *gay-gee-guy*. ...*go-goo-gaw*. ... Do you think you have any difficulty saying any of these sounds? ... Let's say *pay-pea-pie*. ... *poe-poo-paw*. ... Didn't you say /b/ instead of /p/?[1] ... Say them again and hear for yourself. ... I only heard the /b/ sound; so you really have to do something to be understood.[2] The vibrator doesn't help you to make the /p/ sound. That is a voiceless plosive. You shaped your lips for /p/ but it came out /b/,

[1] It is as necessary to develop pressure for the voiceless plosives in using the artificial larynx as it is in esophageal speech. The vibrator works only for the vowels. Practice on the voiceless plosives will develop better articulation with the instrument.

[2] Have the patient practice the vowels with /b/ and /p/, /d/ and /t/ and /g/ and /k/. He should feel how much difference there is in the formation of the voiceless sounds, as in *pay, pea, pie*, etc.

as far as the listener was concerned. Say /p/ without the instrument. ... You have to compress air in your mouth behind the tongue before you can make a /p/. There is no lung air to help you, so it's very important that your sound be heard when you are using the instrument. Here's how to build up the action. Say without the instrument: *pay-pay-pay.* ... Good. With the vibrator, you first say the /p/ and then press the knob for the vowel. Try it. ... Do it this way: start saying *pay-pay* and keep it up for three or four times, then suddenly press the knob. ... That brought out some good /p/ sounds. This will make a contrast between /p/ and /b/. Say *bay-pay.* ... On the first word, the vibrator should have started just before or as you said the /b/. On the second one, you should have delayed the vibrator while you said /p/ and then finished the vowel with the vibrator. I know it's tricky, but practice will make you be a good conversationalist. Say this pair: *boe-poe.* ... *boo-poo.* ... Now do you get the difference?[3]

"Let's do the same action with /d/ and /t/. Without the vibrator, say *tay-tay-tay.* ... Start the vibrator after you say the /t/ in the third *tay.* ... Now, be sure that you vibrate for the /d/ and omit the vibrator for the /t/, saying *day-tay.*" ... Try *dee-tee.* ... *die-tie.* .. *doe-toe.* ... *doo-too.* ... Do the same with *gay-kay.* ... That /k/ was a little harder. Say without the vibrator: *kay-kay-kay.* ... Now say them with the vibrator. ... They all came out *gay-gay-gay.* So you have to say the /k/ before you start the vibrator. Try five of them again and explode the /k/ before you press the knob. ... That was better. Now say these for contrasting /k/ and /g/: *gay-kay.* ... *guy-kye.* ... *go-koe.* ... goo-koo. That's much better articulation.

"Let's compare the /g/ and the /k/ in the final position.[4] Say *beg-beck.* ... Did you get a good explosion on the /k/ or did you just hear

[3] Say these words and be sure that the initial or final voiceless sounds are heard without the vibrator going:

buy-pie; bay-pay; bell-pell; bub-pup; bee-pea; robe-rope; rib-rip; nab-nap; ape-eep; apt-able; apple-pip; pep-pap; pop-pup; pope-lap; lip-wrap; loop-ripe; pile-pill; pool-pail; pop-top; pep up; pepper; paper; popper; whopper; whipper; whoop it up; map it out; mop it up; nip at it; nape of the neck; frying pan; pen pal; pin-up girl; lamb; lump; bump; guppy; puppy; poppy; mopey.

Whip up some apple dumplings; Dip the apples in the caramel pan; Don't buy bubble gum; Get the pop-up popper for the popcorn; Bubble, double trouble.

[4] The /k/ and /g/ sounds require compression of air in the pharnyx and mouth, that is, behind the tongue. The voice for /g/ comes from the vibrator, but the action of the tongue must be made by air compressed behind the tongue. The latter action also is necessary for /k/. It will not be understood unless a definite explosion is produced by releasing the air from behind the tongue.

a /g/ at the end of both words? ... That's right. They were both /g/. Sniff and say *beck*. ... The /k/ must be spoken after you release the knob. Say *beck* again and release after the vowel. ... You got a good one that time. Let's contrast these: *sag-sack*. ... *bag-back*. ... *log-lock*. ... You have to capture air and compress it behind the tongue to make a good /k/. Do these final /k/ sounds: *dock*. ... *lock*. ... *sock*. ... Here's a list for a good workout."[5]

[5] *ruguh-rug; raguh-rag; luguh-lug; begin; begun; ago; again; bag; rag; dig; tag; dog; wag; tug; rug; dogcart; hot dog; cold goat; log wagon; bug in the rug; big gate; to get; log gag; lag sag; hoggy; buggy; boggy; biggest; good guess; rag-rock; rig-rick; log-lock; tag-tack; pic-tock; tick-took; take-key; cup-poke; tack-cat; ticket; took-cook; pick-kick; pick it up; take it back; tack it up; Can Dick take it back? The big, black cat sat on the back step.*

Have the patient work especially on words where a three-letter syllable has a vowel between two plosives. The vibrator is used only on the vowel, e.g., *kick, cot, pot, pet, pit, top, Kate, cat, pat, tack, tick, took, take, pop.*

Unit 53. Working with /z/ and /s/, /ʒ/ and /ʃ/, /dʒ/ and /tʃ/

"The sound of /s/ is often not heard at the ends of words or at the ends of phrases and sentences. Let's say the word *miss* with the instrument. ... Did you hear the /s/? ... I didn't. It sounded more like /z/, because the instrument made the vibrations. Say *miss* without the instrument. ... I heard very little sound at all. That shows two things: the instrument makes the voice for the vowel, but you have to make the /s/ sound by exploding compressed air. Start a hissing sound. ... That is not loud enough to be heard, so we have to build up a good /s/. Let's say, without the instrument, *sisssssss.* I was interested to see whether a vowel would come forth, but I guess you have to depend on the vibrator. Do it this way. Hold the hissing several seconds and at about the middle start the vibrator. ... You got an /s/ first and then a /z/. That is the way you must produce your

/s/ sound. Do it in the reverse. Start a hissing with the knob down and release it halfway through. ... You got /z/ and then /s/. That's the way you end a word with the /s/. Go back to the word *miss*. Use the vibrator for /mi/ and release the knob for the /s/. ... Good. You have it now. Let's contrast the two sounds. Say *his-hiss*. ... *peas-peace*. ... *news-noose*. ... *dies-dice*. ... *eyes-ice*. ... *lace-lease*. ... *The soup is very nice*. ... *Put it on ice, please*. ... *I wish a nice piece of soup bone*. ... Good. Work on the list and be sure to contrast the vibrated /z/ with the voiceless /s/.[1] Practice hissing many times during the day.

"As with /s/, /ʃ/ (*sh*) is not articulated well with the artificial larynx. Round and protrude your lips for /ʃ/ and start the vibrator. ... I didn't hear /ʃ/; I heard /ʒ/ (*zh*) because of the vibration. So you have to work on /ʃ/ without the instrument, again forcing air from the mouth through compression. Say *shshshsh* without the vibrator. ... You got quite a bit of force there, so you should be able to say the /ʃ/ in words without the vibrator being on. Hold the knob down only for /bʊ/ and release it for /ʃ/. Say *bush*. ... *push*. ... *fish*. ... *dish*. ... You will have to work on that quick release; otherwise, there will be no /ʃ/; it will be voiced as in *measure*. So let's get the feeling for that voiced sound. Say *measure*. ... *leisure*. ... *pleasure*. ... That is the sound I was hearing. You must isolate the /ʃ/ sound, that is, say it without the vibrator in action.[2]

"The /tʃ/ sound (*ch*) is made by placing the tongue up for /t/ and saying sharply /ʃ/. Again this is done without the vibrator. Say the word *witch*, but release the vibrator knob for /tʃ/. You are improving your articulation with that sound. Try *catch*. ... *watch*. ... *rich*. ... *down the hatch*. ... Every sound was supported by the vibrator except the /tʃ/, and /h/ was

[1] Practice words:
nose; rose; buzz; bees; easy; has; does; goes; wise; rise; ours; adds; towers; tours; always; husband; webs; tubs; reads; heeds; heads; rubs; homes; seems; drums; gives; leaves; horns; raisins.

same; soon; seat; seed; side; sewed; sop; soup; soap; sap; soon; pencil; pistol; faster; fixer; parcel; miss; kiss; bus; bust; piece; mice; nice; pace; race; traps; wraps; naps; gnats; nets; flakes; flicks; sits; sets; suits; pets; once; dunce; dance; tennis; horse; base.

phase-face; pays-pace; peas-peace; his-hiss; news-noose; dies-dice; eyes-ice; lace-lease; fleas-fleece.

Sift the sand; Pass the beans; Soup's on; Snow sifts under the doors; The sun rises in the east and sets in the west; The cats caught some mice in the cellar; Don't let soap suds get in your eyes; I am sick of working in this mess; Tighten up the loose clothesline; I wish a nice, fresh soup bone; The soup was very nice; More salad, please.

He raises roses with long stems; My cousin, Rose, loves daisies; Bees busily buzzed midst the roses; I saw cows and pigs, dogs and cats, ducks and chickens at the fair; Many won prizes.

[2] *fish; wish; lash; flesh; she; shop; shore; shoot; shake; shine; sunshine; bushes; pushes; wishes; lash-ship; fish-show; push-shall; shoe-shop; ship and shore; shoeshine; ship-shape; The shepherd sheared the black sheep; Shall we go to the seashore?*

omitted.³ Let's compare the voiceless sound to the voiced one, /dʒ/, (dj). Say *witch-wedge. ... latch-lodge. ... chair-jar. ... cherry-Jerry. ... church-surge. ... leach-ledge. ... match-Madge.* ... You must practice in the same manner as with other voiceless sounds; that is, be sure to emphasize the plosive aspect while the vibrator is not running. In the word *ledge*, all sounds are voiced; in *leach*, the /tʃ/ must be exploded while the vibrator is off. Watch this as you practice on the words."⁴

³ *watch; catch; which; hatch; each; speech; reach; watch; church; search; match; touch; catch; watch; chop; catch-chick; each-child; watch-Charley; Charley the chipmunk; chit-chat; Chuck, the woodchuck; Chuck it in the hatch; The chickens hatched the chicks.*

⁴ *fudge; judge; budge; orange; giant; joy; jump; jerk; joke; just; gentle; jacket; jealous; pigeon; danger; enjoy; rejoice; James; John; June; July; Jack the Giant; Fetch the fudge; Sludge is in the engine.*

notch-nudge; butcher-badger; catch-cage; match-Madge; which-wedge; cheap-jeep; chip-jip; chin-gin; chill-Jill; chess-Jess; chain-Jane.

Which size of wedge are you using? The butcher and the badger fought for the carcass; One side cheered, the other side jeered; Jill caught a chill at the bridge party; That chunk is a piece of junk; The enemy raids made the general rage.

Unit 54. Working on Pairs: /f/ and /v/, /θ/ and /ð/

"Say *thin*. ... All I heard was *in*. Bite your tongue lightly and blow air over it. ... That means you have to get the air out of the mouth, not from the vibrator. Blow a /θ/ (*th*) and hold it while you start the vibrator. ... You heard the voiced sound, /ð/, So let's distinguish the two sounds. Say *than-thin. ... teeth-teethe. ... ether-either. ... sooth-soothe. ... wreath-wreathe. ... soothe-south.*¹ ... Again, we have the problem of keeping the vibrator down for all sounds except /s/ in *soothe*, but releasing the knob when the voiceless *th* is required.

¹ For *south*, the vibrator should be used only on the vowel. Have the patient practice so that he can hear the /s/ and /θ/ sharply when the vibrator is off.

"Another set of problem sounds: Say *fine-vine. ... save-safe. ... leave-leaf. ... vain-fain. ... dove-duff. ... move-muff. ... grieve-grief. ... thieve-thief. ... vile-file. ... vat-fat. ... veer-fear. ... Doff your hat to the lovely lady. ... Fifty-five forty or fight.*[2] *... He loathed to work on a lathe. ... Be healthy and happy on your birthday. ... They will all drive together to go to Grandfather's for Thanksgiving. ... Ruth held her breath when the dentist filled her teeth. ...* That was much better articulation. Keep up the good work on this list."[3]

[2] The sounds /s/ and /θ/ are done without the vibrator. This requires fast work in alternating it off and on, but that is the only way to insure understandable speech.

[3] Have the patient say these words many times, being sure to release the knob when the words end with a voiceless sound:

soothe-sooth; clothe-cloth; mother-moth; breathe-breath; then-thin; teethe-teeth; bathe-bath; another brother.

The patient should practice delaying the vibration until the /θ/ has been formed:

thank; think; thick; thin; thing; thumb; thunder; thigh; thief; three; through; thread; throat; threat.

The patient should release the knob before finishing the /θ/:

path; bath; south; mouth; cloth; youth; Ruth; Beth; death; breath; earth; worth; month; fourth; fifth; sixth; tenth; He loathed to work on a lathe; Be happy and healthy on your birthday; I think that it is time for Ruth to go South.

Unit 55. Using a Substitute for /ŋ/

"Will you say *sing?* ... Did you have trouble making the /ŋ/ (*ng*) sound? ... That's because your soft palate is kept raised to produce esophageal speech. This prevents the sound from being purely nasal. Placing the tongue for /n/ will give you the best approximation for the /ŋ/ sound (Tait and Tait). Say *sing* again; start /s/ without the vibrator and finish

/ ɪŋ / with the vibrator. ... Do the same with *sink*. With it, you use voiceless consonants at the beginning and end. ... Let's say some words: *ring-rink*. ... *sang-sank*. ... *cling, clang*. ... *ring-rang-rank*. ... Work on the list of words and develop a distinct finish to the final consonant."[1]

[1] *sang; sank; sing; ring; swing; swank; coming; going; nothing; something; spring; swinging; cling-clang-clank, ding-dong; As the smithy sang, his hammer went bang, clang, clank; The longer finger hurt the longest; Rings on his fingers, rings on his toes; The monkey rides on the donkey's back; Sing a song of sixpence.*

Normalizing Speech with the Artificial Larynx

Unit 56. Using Emphasis and Pitch Change

"The control knob of this particular larynx that we have been depressing for vibration is also used to obtain increases in pitch and loudness. In this case, it raises the pitch about half an octave. Since pitch and loudness are closely related, we can also use the control knob for placing emphasis on certain words or phrases. This is very fortunate, because the speaker can reduce the monotony of his instrument, and at the same time give emphasis and meaning to his conversation. We'll work on emphasis first. Emphasize the word I emphasize. Notice that I press the knob a bit farther down for it. For example, I might say: *I said, 'don't DO that.'* You press the knob farther on DO. ... The farther down you press the knob, the louder the voice. Say this: *What do you WANT?* ... We can change the emphasis like this: *What do YOU want?* ... *Why did you DO that?* ... *DO come in.* ... *I think it's LOVELY.* ... You did those well. Let's take the old politician's phrase to show emphasis: *NOW is the time.* ... *for ALL GOOD men.* ... *to come to the AID of the PARTY.* ... Say the entire sentence and emphasize the correct words. ... Using this list of phrases, emphasize what you think should be meaningful.[1] Say some of them during the day, whenever you have a little time. Remember,

[1] The capitalized words should be spoken louder:

I said, "DON'T DO that"; What do you WANT? What do YOU want? What TIME is it? What time IS it? DO come in; COME IN, please; I think it is LOVELY, don't YOU? Now is the TIME for all good MEN to come to the AID of the party; FOUR SCORE and seven years ago, our FATHERS brought forth on THIS continent, a NEW NATION, conceived in LIBERTY, and DEDICATED to the proposition, that ALL MEN are created EQUAL.

just press the control knob a little farther to increase pitch and emphasis.

"Let's say the politician's speech again to put some music in the words. When we inflect, we increase the pitch. On the word *now*, we start at the highest pitch and glide down on the next three words.[2] Now is the time for you to be decorating your speech. Instead of having people say that it is monotonous, use pitch changes and emphasis, as though you mean what you say.

"Another way to make your speech more interesting and intelligible is to articulate well. We have already worked on that, but you should practice by exaggerating the lip and tongue movements. This conveys the impression of talking louder. One of the best practices is to exaggerate while you are counting from 21 to 100. Many of the important consonants will thus be made more intelligible. Every morning, remember to count by exaggerating the sounds of *t, th, f, k, s, n* and *tw*. You can do this by lip whispering and also with the instrument."

Unit 57. Blending Syllables

"We don't say words exactly as we read them. We don't pronounce and separate syllables as they are spelled. We blend final consonants of syllables with the initial vowels of the following syllables. We also blend the last sound of a word with the first sound of the following word. This is very convenient for the person who uses the artificial larynx. For example, will you say the expression: *black and white?*[1] ... Say it again and notice what you do with the /k/ in *black.* ... You said *bla-kand-white.* say it that way. ... Here's another one: *hang-i-tup.* ... Say it faster and notice that the /t/ blends with *up.* ... Say this one: *se-ti-tup.*[2] ... Say *fik-sit.* ... *Bac-kup to the curb.* ... Get the idea? Try some two-syllable words: *spin-*

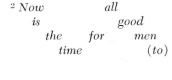

[2] Now   all
    is   good
      the   for   men
        time   (to)

                aid   par
    come the of
to   to   the   ty.

[1] Print it on paper or on the blackboard.

[2] Some speakers might say the two /t/'s in the middle syllable.

ning. ... rum-bling. ... We would li-kour house to be pain-ted in bla-kand white. ... Bring home so-mi-scream. ... Hel-p(h)im ta-kold o-fit. ... Mo-las-ses runs slowly whe-nit's cold. ... Work out the blends in a paragraph. Practice on these words."[3]

Unit 58. Developing Phrasing and Pauses

"Fluency is an important aspect of understandable speech. This means that you keep the sound flowing, but stop at logical points in your conversation. You pause for one or more reasons: to breathe or to think about what you are to say next. You may pause deliberately to give your audience time to think about what you said. However, when you are actually speaking, your words should flow steadily, that is, without hesitation, except for meaning. Then you slow up or speed the rate, as you wish. Say the politician's phrase without stopping for pauses and at one uniform pitch. ... Your artificial larynx stopped at times when you were still talking, and kept going when you paused to get your breath. Divide the sentence into phrases at points where one thought is complete, and notice how much better it sounds. Say it this way: *Now is the time. ... for all good men. ... to come to the aid. ... of the party. ...* Now, say the entire sentence but release the control knob at the point for pausing. ... Then quickly press it when you start the next phrase. ... Your speech was much more pleasant and the thoughts stood out prominently. They are perceived better and understood better. If you notice people who are lecturing, they often pause so long that it is unbearable.[1] Either they want the idea to sink in, or they are thinking about their next idea. Don't be afraid to pause for a definite amount of time, but release the control knob when you are silent.

"The Gettysburg Address is excellent for

[3] *Knuc-kle down to an en-thral-ling task; Ha-s(t)en home for your les-son; Hel-p(h)im ta-kold o-fit; We would li-kour house to be pain-ted in bla-kand-white; Mo-las-ses runs slow-ly whe-nit's cold; Co-min for so-mi-scream.*

[1] Some people use *uh* so many times that their speech is annoying. We heard one instrument user who kept his vibrator going lightly while he hesitated and said "Uh." Some esophageal speakers unconsciously use *uh* as they did before surgery to pause to think what they will say next. This is, incidentally, a good index of naturally recovered speech habits.

making pauses because there are so many thoughts expressed in short phrases. We will say it with one phrase at a time: *Four score and seven years ago. ... our fathers brought forth on this continent. ... a new nation. ... conceived in liberty. ... and dedicated to the proposition. ... that all men are created equal. ...* Now, say it again and pause briefly after each phrase. Get the feeling of the long time, the new nation, the dedication and the equality of men. ... That was an excellent delivery. You have come a long way since we started. I would suggest that you mark off a paragraph of someone's speech that is published in the newspaper. Then deliver it as though you meant everything you said.

"You should remember a few things about your laryngectomy. You should always keep the appointments with your surgeon for rechecks. About the time that you think your batteries are weakening, get a new one so that you always have one on hand. Some men have two complete instruments, keeping a working model for an emergency. Keep it in good working order so that you can always communicate on demand. Meanwhile, perhaps you will be thinking about the possibility of trying to learn esophageal speech. We'll be glad to help you start. "

PARALLEL SPEECH TRAINING WITH THE ARTIFICIAL LARYNX AND ESOPHGEAL SPEECH

We have presented ways and means of helping the laryngectomee to regain communication by learning esophageal speech or by learning to use the artificial larynx. The advantages of the systems are well known and have already been discussed. In recent years, practically all therapists of postlaryngectomy speech have aimed at the production of esophageal speech. (Training laryngectomees to speak with the artificial larynx has not been encouraged.) We have already discussed some of the advantages of using the artificial larynx. It sharpens the accuracy of the patients' articulators and increases the intelligibility of their speech (Diedrich and

Youngstrom; Snidecor). Other advantages could be obtained if the patient were given the opportunity to use both systems of instruction. Therefore, we present a plan for giving parallel instruction in the use of the artificial larynx and in the use of esophageal speech.

Mutual Dividends from Parallel Instruction

An immediate mutual dividend from the use of instruments for both the teacher and the patient is that it permits an easy exchange of information and instructions between them. This is preferable to wasting many minutes and building mutual tensions because the clinician cannot understand the patient and finally requests him to write down what he said. Another mutual advantage is the acquisition of certain speech sounds used with the artificial larynx which may assist in or stimulate the production of esophageal speech sounds. More about this will be said shortly.

Another dividend is the probability of an earlier acquisition of either type of communication by one or the other method. It is certain that if the patient is promptly relieved of the vicious emotional conditions of fear and uncertainty about the loss of speech and its serious consequences, he will more eagerly seek speech recovery.

Ultimately, one or the other type of communication will appear to give the speaker a more intelligible and pleasing reception by his audience. If he acquires esophageal speech as his most reliable means of talking, he will still have the assurance that the use of an instrument will always be available for difficult situations. If he uses the instrument, he will not have any thoughts about his teacher having failed to give him esophageal speech. He also will have had the instruction that should insure high intelligibility and acceptability of speech with an instrument. Finally, he may continue to work on esophageal speech until he acquires good ability in its use, provided that he has the determination to persist.

Several forms of instruction are available for the dual program. The speech clinician can request the patient to imitate a given sound, syllable or phrase, first with the artificial larynx and second with esophageal speech, or vice versa. We have found this successful only in some situations when an exact comparison of the production of the same sound with each speech method was needed. But, generally, the better production was to work for a period of thirty minutes with the instrument, and after a short rest period, to work with the esophageal speech for thirty minutes.*

The question may be raised that if the patient finds the use of the instrument much easier than the learning of esophageal speech, he might indicate his preference for it immediately and not be interested in con-

---

*We have had several conversations with Diedrich, who has used the parallel instruction program, and he agrees with the second method. See page 148 of Diedrich and Youngstrom.

tinuing a dual program. This situation may be avoided by informing the patient that the dual program is intended to give him the most effective speech possible. No decision can be made until he has had rather extensive instruction in both methods of communication. Likewise, the patient should be told that instruction with both instrument and esophageal speech may make it easier for him to learn certain techniques from each method.

Transferring Acquired Speech Patterns from Instrument to Esophageal Speech

Among the advantages that accrue from a parallel program of instruction in two methods of communication is the possibility of developing esophageal voice by using voiced and voiceless plosive consonants with the artificial larynx. The production of the consonants /b/, /d/ and /g/ requires two different processes: the vibratory action from the instrument or the esophagus for the voiced component of the consonants, and the compression of intraoral-pharyngeal air for the voiceless component. (See Tables 31 and 32 of Diedrich and Youngstrom.) This is a strategic point in the instructional program because the adaptation of the articulators to produce the voiceless plosive component with the instrument may aid in the injection of air for producing esophageal speech. (See pages 141 and 142 of Diedrich and Youngstrom.) The speech clinician will recall the use in this text of the trios of syllables in which the patient was required to glide from the voiced consonant to the voiceless consonant and then to repeat the latter to fixate its production. This transference of the voiceless component of the voiced consonant to the production of the isolated voiceless consonant by gliding from, say, *bah,* to *pah, pah,* has occurred repeatedly in our work with esophageal speakers. Hence, we follow the same procedure with the instrument and with the transfer of production of a given sound from the instrument to esophageal speech. The voiced plosive activity, having already been experienced by the patient with the artificial larynx, may provide stimulation to produce by unconscious adaptation a similar sound in esophageal speech. This may occur with a technique such as the following one:

> Ask the patient to say *too-too-too-too* with the instrument very rapidly. He may get an intraphrase injection into his esophagus. With only a pause, have the patient repeat the series without the instrument; he may actually demonstrate esophageal sound. If this does not occur, the usual routine for developing the esophageal sound is again tried and alternated with the instrument series. The intraphrase injection may appear again.
>
> Our other experience has been that the voiced sounds which are learned first with the artificial larynx, such as the /b/ followed by a demand for production of /p/, may be used to transfer the production of /p/ to esophageal speech; in addition, there is a chance that part of the air pressure will enter

the esophagus. Likewise, the syllable *bah,* with its voiced and voiceless components, may enable the patient unconsciously to say the plosive syllable *pah* with esophageal speech. Since the patient is saying *bah* with the instrument, which produces the vibrations for the voiced component, the patient is forced to produce the vibrations for the voiceless component, /p/, by means of intraoral-pharyngeal pressure. This latter component is the part that is transferred to esophageal speech.

The transference of a speech skill acquired in instrumental speech to esophageal speech may occur spontaneously with or without the patient being aware of how it is done. Eventually he must know how it is done so that he can repeat (fixate) the performance at will in esophageal speech. (See Van Riper on fixation of a new sound.) This technique has by no means been a regular occurrence among our patients. However, some rather perceptive patients have accomplished the transfer when we were having difficulty in developing a given sound with the esophageal speech method. They may have been aided by the fact that pharyngeal and esophageal speakers take longer to say vowels and consonant-vowel combinations than users of the artificial larynx (page 86 of Diedrich and Youngstrom). Hence, use of the artificial larynx first may speed up the production of the same sound in esophageal speech. Thus, we might expect that transference to be more likely to occur if the routine instruction with the instrument for the first half of the session is followed by instruction with esophageal speech in the second half.

Formal Parallel Instruction

Instruction with the instrument should begin with Unit 48. Instruction in esophageal speech in the second half-hour should begin with Units 5 through 7. This arrangement places the voiced sounds used with the instrument parallel with the production of their paired voiceless sounds with esophageal speech instruction. The work with the voiced sounds with the instrument gives the patient the sound of speech at once. The auditory and kinesthetic experience may then stimulate him to produce plosive syllables such as *pah* more easily in the half of the session spent on esophageal speech. After Units 5 through 15 have been completed in esophageal speech and Units 48 through 53 have been completed with the instrument, parallel instruction continues as outlined in the remaining material for each method.

Final Adoption of One Method

The time may come when either the patient or the clinician will question the other about continuing with the dual program. If the patient wishes to use esophageal speech exclusively and the clinician agrees to the request, a decision must be made with regard to the abandonment of the other method. Such a decision can be supported by the progress the patient has made. If the instrument has been helpful in improving articulation in esophageal speech, the clinician might suggest that it be used a bit longer. He may suggest that the patient keep the instrument for use in difficult or noisy situations.

If the patient has not improved rapidly with esophageal speech instruction, the clinician may devote more time to training him with the instrument. However, it is not wise to give up completely; rather, the patient should be urged to continue using both methods, especially because the instrument will sharpen the articulation in esophageal speech.

Meanwhile, it is important that the speech clinician, the laryngologist and members of the family maintain their interest in the patient's progress. They should build up his confidence and his determination to improve in communication. However, the most important attitude for others is to praise the patient for doing a good job of learning how to communicate, regardless of the method that is finally adopted. They should reveal no regret concerning the patient's choice of an instrument. The important goal always is the communication that is most adequate, regardless of the method that is adopted and used.*

* In Table 38 of their book, Diedrich and Youngstrom reported that, among six patients who had used an artificial larynx and later learned esophageal speech, four were above the median speech score of thirty-three esophageal speakers. One had the highest score and three had the third and fourth highest scores. The other two were better than the six lowest-scoring noninstrument users. It would appear that use of the artificial larynx had sharpened their articulation before they learned esophageal speech.

Chapter Eight

LOST CHORD CLUBS AS FACTORS IN REHABILITATION

WHY MANY LARYNGECTOMEES HAVE NOT BEEN TOTALLY REHABILITATED

The failure of as many as 40 per cent of laryngectomees to talk, and the known fact that many of those who communicate by esophageal speech are not wholly intelligible, point to weaknesses in the total rehabilitation services for these people. Suspicion of the ineffectiveness of these services may be raised by asking a few questions:

1. Did the surgeons furnish the Lost Chord Clubs with the names of all laryngectomees for visitations?

2. Were all of the laryngectomees adequately oriented in the pre- and/or postoperative periods?

3. Were all of the laryngectomees visited in the hospital?

4. Were the presentations of the visitants beneficial?

5. Did the spouses of the Auxiliary call on the spouses of the newly laryngectomized persons?

6. If a patient was visited and invited to the Lost Chord Club meetings, why did he not come?

7. If he appeared once, why did he not return a second time?

8. If the visitant and surgeon urged him to begin speech lessons, why did he not take them?

9. If he started speech lessons, why did he not finish them?

10. If he did not learn esophageal speech, why was he not given an opportunity to communicate by use of the artificial larynx?

11. Have all the ways and means of decreasing the percentage of speech failures been made available to the therapists?

12. If they have been available, why have they not been used?

13. Were the teachers of esophageal speech efficiently trained to pursue a broad program of rehabilitation?

14. Are those who are directly involved in the various phases of serving laryngectomees concerned only with bits and pieces of the total program?

15. Has there been a failure in the coordination of the total program by responsible persons or groups?

16. How many professional persons or prominent laryngectomees have conscientiously assumed the responsibility for following the progress of the laryngectomee through the various stages from surgery to ultimate, adequate communication and successful social and economic adjustment?

Many of these questions have been answered in earlier chapters of this book. If the suggestions given in connection with these questions are used, many of the weaknesses mentioned above can be corrected.

WHO CAN HELP THE LARYNGECTOMEE?

We have some ideas on the reasons for the low incidence of rehabilitation of laryngectomees. Among these are lack of interest by individuals in the welfare of handicapped persons and inadequate capability or training of the persons or organized groups who do become interested in the problem. We have known few speech pathologists who cared enough to follow through on all of the successive steps of rehabilitation. This is regarded by them as just one small phase of their total pathological field. We also have known others who have not assumed this responsibility at all, although it is available and the need is obvious.

Veterans Administration hospitals and facilities have an excellent opportunity to perform a responsible, complete program of rehabilitation for a selected number of laryngectomees, namely, veterans of the wars. The staffs have unusually strict control of their patients and can program a most comprehensive and intensive training of their patients. They have available not only capable speech clinicians but also all of the ancillary services, psychological, social and economic, for evaluating the patients' problems. They have proved that an intensive program in depth is necessary for successful acquisition of speech.

Speech and hearing centers are also in a good position to carry much larger loads of nonmilitary laryngectomees. The centers are manned by professionally trained persons who have backgrounds not only in speech pathology and audiology but also in educational methods, psychology and in some instances psychotherapy. Likewise, the centers have available, on the staff or within the area, psychologists and social workers who are capable of evaluating the personalities and capabilities of patients who appear to be depressed or incapable of rising above their difficulties. In some cities, the laryngologist utilizes the services of the centers to fulfill his plan to rehabilitate the patient.

There are several hundred *laryngectomized teachers* who are now taking over some of the load of instruction of the ever-increasing numbers of laryngectomees. These teachers, through annual training programs at the institutes, are becoming more efficiently skilled in teaching methods than those who learned to talk without instruction or who were trained by poor instructors. (See chapter 5 for discussion of this problem.)

Lost Chord Clubs are fast becoming an important medium for the more complete planning of rehabilitation of laryngectomees. Under the guidance of their national headquarters, the IAL and the American Cancer Society, the clubs are developing into more capable media for helping the patients. If the clubs are associated with a hearing and speech center, or with speech pathologists from a neighboring university, they become a logical center for rehabilitation (Martin). The centers, as well as the laryngologists, refer the patients to the clubs for purposes of recreational rehabilitation.

The Lost Chord Clubs may have the appearance of a social group; however, they offer the newly laryngectomized person an opportunity to meet many other persons who have been deprived of the larynx. In the process of having a good time, the club members demonstrate to the visitors that they give little appearance of being handicapped, disfigured, depressed or anxious; rather, they appear to be well adjusted and successful in business and in social activities. As the newly laryngectomized person enjoys meeting many good esophageal speakers, he becomes aware of a feeling of relief and anticipation: relief because anxiety is replaced by inner assurance that he is going to like these people, talk, be happy, have friends and dress naturally; anticipation because he is now confident that he will be getting back on the job and earning a living again. Depression and anxiety usually fade away with each step to clearer speech and to a desire to have a social life like other laryngectomees.

HOW LOST CHORD CLUBS HELP THE LARYNGECTOMEE

Readjustments Through Contact with the Lost Chord Club

Referral to a Lost Chord Club does not mean that some club member will take the patient in hand and inquire into his psychological and domestic problems, although some clubs have given the impression that this and other types of services are available. No club member, however successful he is in business or as a speech teacher, has the authority to perform services that are ordinarily practiced by professionally trained persons. To be sure, they demonstrate enthusiasm and encouragement, and they prove that they have overcome their own handicaps. In addition, they demonstrate adequate speech.

Martin clearly states the purpose of the club when he writes:

The most serious hindrances to prompt and complete rehabilitation of the laryngectomee are mental depression and lowering of morale. For these disorders, one of the best remedies is social contact with other laryngectomees in various stages of rehabilitation. For this reason, wherever as many as three or four laryngectomees can be brought together, they should be encouraged to form a club, entirely independent of the teaching unit.

Martin's statement confirms our belief that much ado has been made over the possible need for psychiatric guidance of laryngectomized persons. The general consensus among professional persons who have maintained interest in the welfare of laryngectomees, and who have talked casually or formally about postoperative reactions, is that most of the patients are able to make satisfactory adjustments without psychiatric aid. We have learned from personal interviews with laryngologists that they have rarely had to refer patients to a psychiatrist because of pending laryngectomy. Damsté knew of only one among his patients who was truly depressed. According to laryngologists, an occasional patient may be so distraught that he is referred to a psychiatrist to explore the possibility of serious traumata. However, the psychiatrist usually finds that it is only necessary to handle the fears of the patient so that he becomes able to accept the surgeon's verdict.

In view of these findings and opinions, we believe that the Lost Chord Clubs can be the avenue for the easiest and quickest readjustments by these people. Hence, outlined below are suggestions that large or small groups of laryngectomees may use to help themselves and their fellow members to make satisfactory return to their milieu.* We believe that if the clubs can succeed in bringing more and more of the laryngectomees into the club activities, a larger proportion of successfully rehabilitated persons will be reported.

Services of the Clubs

The 145 clubs that belong to the IAL function under a charter that requires annual renewal. The purpose of the renewal is to cause the club officials to review the important standards under which they function. These are designed to guide each club in the maintenance of an effective and active program of service to the laryngectomees of its area. The club officials must agree to cooperate with the medical profession, some of whom are on the club's Board of Directors. Each club shall cooperate with quasi-medical agencies and public, private or governmental organizations, who may assist in the total rehabilitation of laryngectomees. In addition, the club must cooperate with the American Cancer Society

---

* We still have an unhappy feeling that some of the 40 per cent of patients who are unsuccessful in speech may have been the ones who needed psychiatric advice.

and/or other cancer-fighting organizations in the overall fight against cancer. They shall strive to provide for, or arrange for, transportation of laryngectomees to training centers for teaching speech. In order to insure an effective program, the clubs must operate under a committee structure that provides professional advice, visitations to patients, safety and first aid, public education and rehabilitation.

The Professional Advisory Committee

Inasmuch as continuous responsibility for rehabilitation of the laryngectomized person rests with surgeons (Martin), one or more of them should be members of the committee. Likewise, the executive director of the local or sponsoring speech and hearing center, or a speech pathologist designated by the center, should serve on the committee. A genuine contribution to the committee can be made by a representative of the local cancer society. Several businessmen can make valuable contributions to the efficient administration of the club. Finally, one or more members of the club will fill out the membership of the committee.

In order to oversee the rehabilitation of laryngectomees, the committee has the supervision of ethical practices and policies of all committees of the club. It approves or authorizes the writing of literature that may be used in the club programs. It may approve distribution of literature and use of films furnished by the local and state units of the American Cancer Society and of similar organizations. The committee sets policies on the nature and extent of counsel and service that other committees and members may give to newly laryngectomized persons and to the public; it also plans for the growth of the club's activities and designates members and committees to work out the details of the plans.

The Patient Visitation Committee

The members of this committee are appointed by the Board of Directors because they have good speech, are well adjusted and well dressed and have had successful postoperative employment. The visitants operate under instructions that are laid down by annual workshops over which a surgeon presides. They discuss problems encountered in making visitations and in turn the surgeon presents any misunderstandings that may have occurred between the surgeons and the visitants. One important rule is strictly observed: no visitation shall be made to any patient without the formal permission of the surgeon. The surgeon also must approve the literature that the visitant might leave with the patient, and there must be general agreement on the content of the conversation. Visitants are not permitted to discuss finances or medical problems. They are required to advise the patients to ask their surgeon.

A coordinator's telephone number is furnished to the offices of all surgeons. This person may be the wife of one of the club members. She receives the requests from the surgeon, who gives the patient's name and room number in the hospital. The coordinator then telephones visitants until she obtains promises from three of them to visit the patient. She designates one of them to take the kit of materials that is to be given to the patient. The kit consists of a magic slate; an envelope of gauze bibs which are made by volunteers of the American Cancer Society; the booklets *Helping Words* and *Laryngectomees at Work*, which are published by IAL and the American Cancer Society, and the club's welcome pamphlet. If the patient can only speak a foreign language, the coordinator endeavors to send a visitant who speaks that language.

The surgeon's request is the signal for the entire visitation program to begin. This has already been presented in the early pages of this book; hence, we will only state here that the wife of a laryngectomee may call upon the wife of the patient. Also, if the patient is a female, a female laryngectomee may call upon her. (The contents of all visitants' remarks are to be found in the early pages of this book.) The visitants send the chairman of the committee a card which contains data about the patient and the date of the visit. The visitant is required to inform the coordinator if he was unable to make the visit, so that another member can be assigned to the visitation.

The Membership Committee

The enthusiastic work of the visitants gains the attention and interest of the newly laryngectomized person. The Membership Committee endeavors to keep active this attention and interest. The following steps are taken to persuade the patient to become an active worker in the club:

1. The new patient is sent a letter of welcome and an invitation to the next meeting of the club.

2. The spouse from the Auxiliary who had visited the patient's wife earlier now urges her to be sure to arrange for her husband to come to the club meeting.

3. The male or female visitant (a laryngectomee) will also remind the patient to come to the next club meeting.

4. Some clubs have a transportation committee which directs drivers to bring the various members to the meeting.

The Greeters

When the patient makes his first visit to the club, the Greeters welcome him. They are charged with the following duties:

1. Greet the patients and their spouses as they come in.
2. Record attendance and the names of visitors.
3. Make a list of new members and visitors to be given to the president, who will introduce them.
4. Give the new member a questionnaire to fill in about his hobbies, his wife's name, whether he will return to work and if not, why not. This report will be studied by the Rehabilitation Committee.
5. Pin a ribbon on him to indicate that he is a new member so other members will greet him.
6. Present the new member with a kit that contains (a) an emergency pocket card that warns safety officials that he is a laryngectomee, (b) an emergency windshield sticker to notify safety officials in case of emergency, (c) a copy of the club's recent bulletin and (d) a copy of the *IAL News*.
7. Obtain a correct record of his name, address, zip code and telephone number for the use of the mailing service, for the name badge and for the *IAL News*.

The Greeters make a motion during the meeting to accept him as a member.

Public Education and Information Committee

Future laryngectomees and the general public benefit from the activities of this committee, which obtains appearances on television and interviews on the radio. Aided by the publicity staff of the local cancer society, the members lecture and give demonstrations with films on the dangers of smoking and its relation to cancer of the larynx. Motion pictures and slides tell vividly the story of the people who breathe through a hole in the neck. One group of speakers talked to 16,240 children and adults in fifty-four schools and fifteen other organizations in one year.

Speakers are trained by assisting in the distribution of pamphlets and by meeting the public. Slow, timid speakers soon request an opportunity to say something. Speaking only a few words at their first attempts, they become fluent speakers by the end of the season. Their own problems fade away as they regain-self-confidence, which makes them eager to perform public services and duties they would have firmly avoided in the past as normally speaking persons.

First Aid and Safety Committee

If a man with a hole in his neck collapses on the street, few people will treat him differently from someone without such a hole. When hospital personnel prepared to treat a man who was brought in after injury in an automobile accident, they found a hole in his neck. Not knowing what to do, they sent him to a hospital located fifty miles away. Another laryngectomee was admitted for treatment of pneumonia. An attendant inserted the feeding tube into the stoma. The patient slapped it away. After two more attempts and a consultation with a superior, she put it in his nose. These incidents point to the great need for educating the public and safety and first-aid personnel on how to recognize and give first aid to laryngectomized persons.

Members are trained to become skilled at demonstrating methods of reviving heart and accident victims, especially laryngectomees. They are formed into teams, with a physician always one of the members, to present first-aid methods. Slides are used to supplement the demonstrations. These have been prepared by the Committee on Safety of the IAL.

The committee may make a study of working conditions that might injure laryngectomees. It can begin action when a member states that he has lost his job because of working conditions. It can investigate the credibility of the employer's excuse for the discharge, or call upon industrial hygiene specialists to evaluate the problem in terms of possible damage to a person who breathes through a stoma.

> A post office worker was recommended for early retirement because the physician decided that the dust in the assorting room would damage the patient's lungs. The physician was told that laryngectomees are employed in post offices in other cities of the nation. Nevertheless, the man was not reemployed. Perhaps a different approach to the physician or to a higher authority would have brought better results.

> A laryngectomee was disemployed by a local railroad physician because a fireman's job would be a hazard to the laryngectomee and to the railroad. Arrangements were made by one of the club physicians for the employee to be examined in another city by the chief surgeon. The latter decided that since the work consisted largely of turning valves and watching dials, it was not hazardous to the employee. In this case, arguments with the local physician would have been fruitless (Fig. 13).

These cases indicate the need that commands consideration of ways and means of protecting the stoma from toxic fumes and particulate matter. (See Gardner 1964 for hazards to laryngectomees in industry.)

Although some masks have been built specifically for neck breathers, and older models have been modified for them, none have been successful in protecting all laryngectomees from all industrial gases. (See Gardner 1964 for information on the effect of toxic gas and chemical products on laryngectomees and for recommendations for protection.) The committee should continue to research for improvements in gas masks for neck breathers, and to urge research departments of industries to continue to

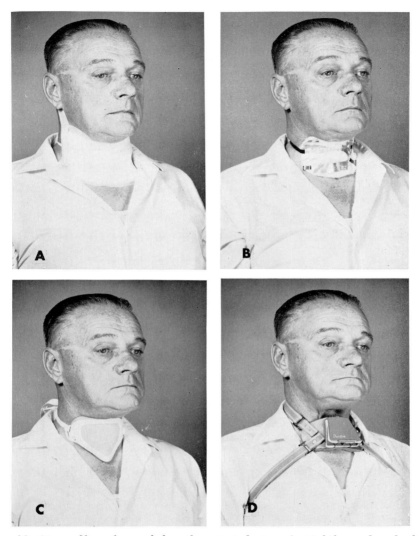

Figure 13. Stoma filters for neck breathers in industry: *A.* Multilayered pad of gauze taped to skin. *B.* Martindale Protective Nose Mask adapted to stoma breathing (Martindale Electric Company). *C.* Nose mask adapted to cover stoma. *D.* Filter part of Dustfoe No. 66 Respirator attached to foam rubber with opening for stoma breathing (Mine Safety Appliances Company). (*Courtesy of American Medical Association*)

search for better methods of protection. The committee therefore may very well work with those who are interested in air pollution.

Rehabilitation Committee

This committee has two subcommittees, one for reemployment problems and the other for promoting speech recovery for all laryngectomees. The committee as a whole may be composed of several club members, an industrial physician, a personnel officer of a corporation and a representative of the local Bureau of Vocational Rehabilitation. The subcommittee on speech therapy may be composed of a speech pathologist, a laryngectomized esophageal speech teacher who has had training at an institute for teaching esophageal speech and several members of the Lost Chord Club.

The duties of the subcommittee on speech could be:

1. Arrange for acceptable speech therapy for every member.

2. Set up standards or levels of speech achievement for members.

3. Encourage all members to achieve higher levels in communication.

4. Have annual awards for the greatest gains in speech fluency and intelligibility, the evaluation being given by impartial speech clinicians.

5. Endeavor to locate nonspeakers in the community in order to obtain speech therapy for them. This work should be done in cooperation with the Membership Committee.

6. Recommend use of the artificial larynx early for those members who have demonstrated inability to communicate adequately with esophageal speech. The criteria for this requirement should be set up by the club. Such criteria may be found in Chapter 4.

7. Recommend a hearing aid for a spouse whose hearing loss thwarts efforts of the esophageal speaker to be heard.

8. Recommend that patients whose speech is affected by hearing loss wear a hearing aid for their own comfort as well as that of others.

9. Recommend use of an amplifier on the telephone for those whose weak voices otherwise cannot be heard well.

10. Furnish group speech therapy at monthly meetings of the club and at frequent intervals between meetings, if no other facility is available.

11. Arrange with local and state units of the American Cancer Society to support financially the employment of a speech clinician or a trained laryngectomee to give group and/or individual speech lessons to newly laryngectomized persons, such lessons to be furnished without cost to the patients. (In Ohio, the state division of the American Cancer Society has arranged speech instruction for all laryngectomees in the state at six university speech and hearing centers. The branch offices of the U.S. Department of Vocational Rehabilitation may likewise furnish free speech lessons to patients they find feasible for rehabilitation.

12. Local clubs may consult the chairman of the Speech Standards Committee of the IAL for the standards of speech instruction that they should adopt.

Group therapy for laryngectomees has advantages that are not present in speech therapy for one person. This is especially important if the group is mixed, that is, has patients who have attained different levels of achievement, or who may or may not be seriously depressed. In fact, the group may consist of only the members of the club, receiving their regular speech stimulation. New patients should be included in the group, but they should not be forced to make any speech effort until they are ready emotionally and until they can produce an esophageal sound.

Mutuality of problems, where everyone in the group has had loss of speech with resultant emotional disturbances, enables the members to realize that they are not alone in their misfortunes (Damsté; Martin 1963). It helps them to help each other to overcome the sense of being handicapped (Laguaite). The sympathetic atmosphere prevents patients who are, or think they are, badly disfigured, for example, or who are especially sensitive over communication disabilities, from withdrawing from their friends and business acquaintances. Group speech therapy helps them to overcome their self-pity, fears, sense of guilt and disgust over their appearance. (Gardner 1966; M.C.L. Greene; Nahum and Golden). Friendly encouragement by well-adjusted members gives others the determination to regain their lost speech skills (Locke). Their self-confidence may be restored and their ego bolstered as they become proficient in communication. Those who live alone or feel socially ostracized soon realize that they need the companionship of others (Lanpher 1967). Indeed, if they are willing to work with the speech group, they may become involved in the competitive exercises with others, forget their troubles and rejoice in their new triumphs. The following is a good illustration of the type of change that may come from group speech therapy:

> A middle-aged female laryngectomee had isolated herself from friends and all community activities. She was persuaded to visit a Lost Chord Club, where she observed laryngectomees having group speech therapy and enjoying speech games. Finally becoming aware of what she had been doing to herself, she decided to visit a social club which she had abandoned. She was amazed at the warm welcome that the members gave her. Later, she became an officer and thenceforth immersed herself in many community affairs.

It has been most interesting and enlightening to see the transformation of laryngectomees, especially those who appeared to have little opportunity to improve their social life. After they had the joy of participating with others in speech projects, they joined hands to help newly laryngectomized persons. Others rose to the ranks of leadership as officers in neighborhood organizations. Some, who had never given a speech before a group, became able public speakers and ran for political offices. They reached greater heights than they would have with their original, normal speech.

The subcommittee on reemployment may be composed of a personnel officer of a corporation, a representative from the Bureau of Vocational Rehabilitation, a physician specializing in industrial hygiene and several members of the club. Retaining a job or obtaining one after having been discharged because of a so-called handicap requires the support of the committee. Damsté reported that 16 per cent of his laryngectomees in The Netherlands lost their jobs. Gardner (1964) reported that 28 per cent of laryngectomees lost or changed jobs. In 1965, Ranney found that 24 per cent changed or lost jobs. About 18 per cent were fired, 4 per cent were demoted and 2 per cent resigned. In 1966, Gardner reported that 55 per cent of laryngectomized women who had worked before surgery returned to the same jobs after surgery that is, 45 per cent did not return to their jobs. A more recent report by Diedrich and Youngstrom indicated that only 56 per cent had the same job they had before surgery; 23 per cent retired because of surgery and the rest remained unemployed.

The statistics just mentioned should stimulate the committee to evaluate the causes of job loss. Some of the reasons that may be explored are those given by employers when they discharged workers (Gardner 1964):

1. Endangering the lives of fellow employees.
2. Poor speech, especially during an emergency.
3. Age and physical condition of the laryngectomee.
4. Conditions of the job which might affect the health of the worker.
5. Work habits and attitudes of the worker.

Employees, however, have their own opinions about the loss of their jobs. Ranney found that only ninety-one of 239 discharged or demoted laryngectomees agreed with the action taken by the employers. Fifty-four believed that they could have handled their jobs as efficiently as they did before surgery. Likewise, ninety-three of 192 laryngectomees who were discharged said that they were still capable of doing other jobs at their places of employment. Among Gardner's group of thirty-three dis-charged laryngectomees, all except one stated that employers were not well informed about the true capabilities of laryngectomees and about practical methods of rearranging their employment. They argued that they were the same men as before surgery, with the same abilities to use their heads, their eyes, their feet, their backs and their hands. They com-plained bitterly that other employees who had heart disease or were epileptic were not discharged. Figure 14 shows some of the many different types of jobs that can be held by laryngectomees.

Although the Lost Chord Club cannot perform the service of finding jobs for disemployed laryngectomees (many agencies are available to do this), it can assist them in retaining or regaining their employment status in three different ways. The committee can promote a general educational program for employers on the importance of retaining laryngectomized persons. This can be done by speaking at assemblies of employers or employment personnel. The attitudes and superstitions of employers and employees can be changed considerably by this kind of activity. Since the start of the "Employ the Handicapped" programs, which have been sponsored by both government and private organizations, employers have been more receptive to arguments on behalf of laryngectomees and employees more readily accept them.

A second method of helping the disemployed is to make advance preparations to prevent the employee's discharge. Martin (1963) has made the following suggestion:

> In such situations, I believe that if the surgeon himself gets in touch with the employer by telephone, it becomes almost impossible for the employer to decline to cooperate. Psychologically, the opportunity is better before operation rather than after. . . . In my experience there is as much heart and sympathy in big business as in any social service or welfare agency, and what is even of greater importance, more power to act immediately and effectively.

In lieu of the surgeon's telephone call, a member of the club may visit the patient's personnel officer or employer to explain the situation and to obtain assurance that the company will gladly have him return to his job when he is fully recovered.

A third method of helping the disemployed patient is to learn as much as possible about his intention to return or not to return to work. Much information may be obtained from the questionnaire the new member fills out when he first joins the club. If the patient is depressed or discouraged or doubtful about his future employment, the surgeon may be asked to indicate any physical weakness resulting from surgery which might prevent the patient from carrying on the same job. Likewise, a social worker may be requested to search for sources of worries or doubts in the patient, and even to inquire into conditions at home. Having favorable information from these sources, the committee will work with more assurance that the patient probably will lose his anxieties through participation in club activities. The chances, then, are good that he will decide to return to his job.

If the patient is able, he should be advised to get back on the job as soon as possible—of course, with the surgeon's permission. He should not

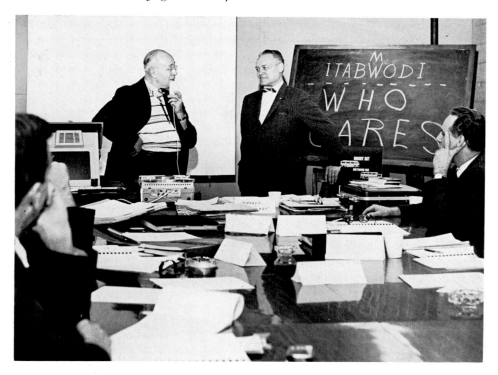

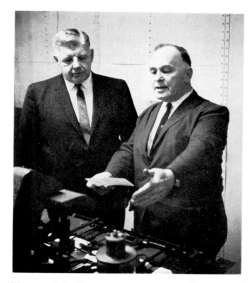
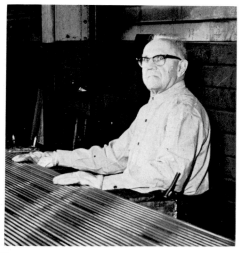

Figure 14. Laryngectomees working at different occupations: *A.* Laryngectomee as director of training (*standing right*). *B.* Salesman displaying office equipment to purchasing agent; both men are laryngectomees. *C.* Laryngectomee operating electric furnace at age 74.

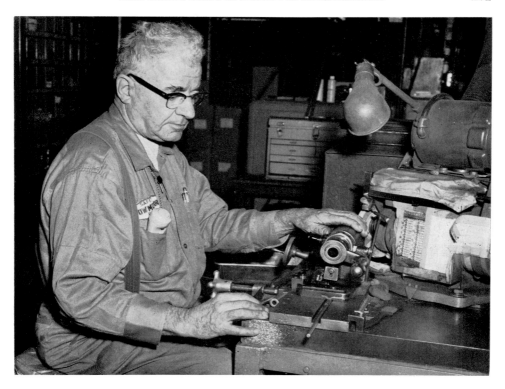

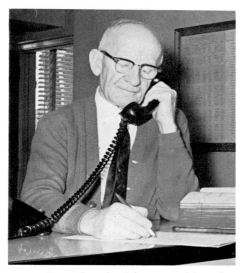

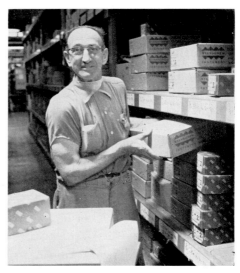

D. Tool grinder; he has no problem from air particles entering stoma. Note electric larynx, which he must use in noisy place. *E*. Records clerk in coroner's office; he uses three telephones, asks about 500 questions daily and records answers in book shown. *F*. Shipping clerk; lifts packages as heavy as ninety pounds.

wait to acquire adequate speech. The employer should be given the impression that speech will come later. In some situations, employers insist that patients not report to work until they can talk, whereas other employers urge them to return regardless of their ability to talk. The patient can always communicate with the artificial larynx when it is necessary; as time goes on, he will use esophageal speech more than he does the instrument. Some employers have told patients that they prefer esophageal speech and have encouraged them to develop it.

Another reason why the patient should return to the job quickly is to forestall any ideas the employer may have to replace him. This has happened numerous times; when the employee did not return for several months, the employer could not wait. At least the patient's early return will give him the opportunity to prove to the employer that he can do the job as efficiently as before. Furthermore, if he does not succeed on the old job, he will be less likely to be dropped; rather, he may be transferred to another job.

An important word of caution is given the patient who has been transferred to a job that results in a lower salary. He is warned not to become angry over the demotion, or to resign, as he may lose the rights and privileges of employment, which include pensions, insurance, medical compensations and bonuses. Unfortunately some laryngectomees express their dissatisfaction and resign, losing advantages they have accumulated over the working years.

An excellent example of the self-confidence and determination that enables a laryngectomee to overcome the attitudes or doubts of the employer is revealed by the following story:

> A laryngectomee had been a training sales supervisor in a large organization. When he returned to work after his laryngectomy, he was given a desk job. His superiors were surprised to hear him talking over the intercommunication system. He next insisted that they should try him out on work that involved talking to people. He demonstrated that he could talk to groups with his new type of speech. He next asked if he could go back on sales training, as an assistant. He wanted to prove that he could do as well as he had done before. Eventually, he was given back his former directorship and has kept the job without any doubts by his employers that he would fail.

The Women's Auxiliary

The wives of laryngectomized men can make substantial contributions to the recreational activities of the club by supervising the preparation and serving of refreshments for the social hour after the business meeting. The wives knit or crochet bibs for sale to the members. They also raise funds for sending members to the conventions, or for the expenses of refreshment, and for purchasing equipment that may be helpful to the members.

The wives have a committee that has separate sessions with the wife of a new laryngectomee. The committee advises her on family adjustments to speed her husband's learning of speech. The following suggestions have been gleaned from such sessions and are offered for the benefit of wives and teachers of postlaryngeal speech:

If not already arranged, the spouse should plan for the patient's first visit to the speech therapist as soon as the surgeon orders it. She must give him the impression that this is a routine procedure, not to be delayed. She should encourage him to practice as frequently as the teacher suggests. It will be helpful to prepare an atmosphere for practice by setting up a schedule of periods and arranging a chair and table for his notes and books. She also should remind him that he will get great benefit from the meetings of the Lost Chord Club.

Emphasis should be placed on the importance of being patient with the husband's speech growth. It takes time to develop an entirely new form of speech. Fluency comes only after esophageal speech is well developed. She should remind him that it is better to say one-syllable words with one breath than to say several phrases or a sentence that are not intelligible; furthermore, people will more easily understand him.

Although the wife may anger him (some husbands resent "being told" by their wives) by insisting that he turn off the television and get busy, she should be firm about this and tell him that only her love for him makes her so stubborn.

When he has learned a few words, the wife should encourage him to say single words in conversation, and always to answer by voice for *Yes, No, Ok, Hi, Bye, Fine, I am fine,* etc. He should learn additional household words every day.

After he attempts conversation, she should pay close attention to what he is saying. She should stop what she is doing and watch his lips. She should not, however, lean forward intently with mouth open or repeat words with her lips. This causes him to become anxious and tense and fear that he is not improving. She should not irritate him by saying that she understands when he is only half through the sentence, or by nodding her head. It is always better to tell him frankly that she did not understand and to ask him to repeat what he said. If it is obvious that he is having difficulty with a key word, the wife should not hesitate to tell him to write it down. (This difficulty would be avoided by having an artificial larynx for such difficulties.) However, the time may come when she can say: "Go on and try it again: I can wait." This encourages eventual success.

When he is improving rapidly, he should be encouraged to talk longer and at more frequent intervals. The time will come for him to be encouraged to read aloud both prepared and unfamiliar material. Praise him for each step gained. His old friends should be asked to visit him so that he can talk with them and overcome timidity. The most important discovery for the patient is that people will accept him with his new voice.

The social hour is the peak of the club meeting because the new members meet many of the older members, who greet them effusively. After such an evening, it will be only the most uninterested person, or one without insight into his own problems or into his future, who will not return for succeeding club sessions. The stimulation that the wife receives from the counseling of the wives greatly encourages her with the thought that it will not be long before the family will be back in the old routine, with the husband back on the job and money coming in to furnish the family with the necessities of life.

The Transportation Committee

Members who do not drive or are too old to drive, and others who cannot drive in the dark, need some help in being transported to the club meetings. Members make a special point of bringing new members so that they will acquire an early interest in the club activities. The committee divides the city and its suburbs into areas according to zip codes. A driver is assigned to each zone. Members who do not wish to participate in administrative activities can assume the task of transporting members.

CASE HISTORIES

Case 1. Male, 57 years old; complained of hoarseness and difficulty in swallowing. Diagnosis was cancer on the entire length of the left vocal fold and extending around the anterior commissure to the right vocal fold.

Patient was seen preoperatively for speech instruction. Motion picture, *New Voices*, was shown and literature given. He was taught to swallow air· and belch it back, after using carbonated beverage (year 1957).

Surgery was performed for a total laryngectomy and left radical dissection. Speech clinician visited the patient daily. On the sixth postoperative day, the surgeon ordered visitors from the local Lost Chord Club. The feeding tube was removed on the same date. The patient was discharged on the fourteenth postoperative day.

Two weeks later: Patient returned for first postoperative checkup. Was referred to speech clinician. Lesson devoted to injecting air by the swallow technique. After the third lesson in one week, the patient was unable to make an esophageal sound. He did not return for lessons.

Sixth month checkup. Patient again referred to speech therapist. The patient had a very strong, deeply pitched esophageal voice. The sound was of short duration so that speech was frequently interrrupted for air-charge. When he phonated, a large round bulge about the size of a golf ball was seen to vibrate in the neck to the right of the esophageal line. When a finger was pressed on it, the vibration was felt but it did not interfere with the phonation. The impression of the surgeon was that a section of the wall of the esophagus had become weakened and resulted in the formation of a pocket. However, the true pseudoglottis was still located at the top of the esophagus. The patient was now trained to extend the phonation in order to get more fluency.

One month later. The patient was able to produce five or six syllables on one phonation. He had become fluent enough to be able to sell house-to-house items.

Case 2. Male, 52 years old. Patient complained of a hoarse voice but without pain. He had been an inveterate smoker. Diagnosis was cancer on both vocal folds. Preoperative speech therapy was devoted to the swallow-belch, aided by carbonated beverage.

Surgery was simple laryngectomy. He made good recovery and was referred on the seventeeth postoperative day for speech therapy, having left the hospital on the tenth postoperative day. Therapy was directed toward probing for ability to make an esophageal sound. Patient reported that he had made a burp occasionally after eating a meal in the hospital. After demonstration of injecting air, the patient compressed his lips and made a weak sound. It appeared that he also lifted his tongue at the time he made the air-charge. After several trials, he made very good air expulsions. He counted up to 10, making an injection for each number. He produced some vowels on command, weak but recognizable. On an effort to produce two syllables, the second one was whispered.

One week later. Duration of vowel phonation was two seconds. He could phonate on voiced sounds better than with unvoiced consonants, so we worked on dipthongs and voiced consonants, increasing duration of tone and use of it for two syllables. Likewise, two- and three-word phrases were demonstrated and worked on.

One week later. The patient demonstrated ability to talk in short sentences and phrases of three syllables. Voice was somewhat stronger but faded at ends of phrases and sentences. He appeared to be anxious to keep the voice coming, which resulted in skipped sounds and whispered syllables. We explained that intelligibility was the goal, not speed at this time. We worked on two- and three-syllable phrases until he could maintain phonation to the last sound. He demonstrated increased fluency and intelligibility during these exercises. He did not return for further lessons.

One month later. Patient returned for medical checkup. All was negative but he was referred to the speech clinician. He was a fluent talker but still missed some sounds at the ends of phrases. Was urged to take his time. Voice was adequately loud for a small crowd. He later became president of a Lost Chord Club and the teacher. He was a successful teacher, as witnessed by the pupils he taught.

Case 3. Male patient, 72 years old. He had had a simple laryngectomy thirty months before his visit. He had been taught to swallow air for injection. He had had weekly lessons for over two years. He could only produce one word at a time. He could not initiate a single sound on command; rather he protruded his jaw, compressed his lip, hesitated, then swallowed finally and belched loudly.

Brief experimentation showed that he could easily make an esophageal sound with rapid repetition of *pah*. Plosive syllables *pah, tah* and *kah* were quickly learned. He soon spoke words like *pit, pet, top, and coat.*

Two weeks later. Patient was able to prolong vowels for two seconds. We worked on two-syllable words per injection. After having success with these, we tried three syllables. His voice faded on the last syllable; however, he remarked that this was the first time he had ever said two syllables on one breath. Short phrases and sentences were next given to him, for practice at home.

One month later. Patient talked with short phrases and sentences and stated that he had talked over the telephone for the first time in over two years. Since he played the piano, we emphasized a musical voice, demonstrating it with inflection and emphasis. He did not return for therapy.

Two months later. Patient demonstrated ability to express himself freely and showed none of the hesitancy that was so characteristic of his first behavior. He read the Rainbow passage (Test 7 in Chapter 6) at the rate of 109 words per minute.

Case 4. Demonstrating the whistle technique.

A male, 46 years old, had had a simple laryngectomy four weeks before his first lesson. We demonstrated a clear, sharp whistle with the tiny toy whistle and asked him to try it. After two minutes of experimentation, he developed a sharp, loud whistle, which is a requirement for success. We next urged him to feel for any air moving backward when he blew the whistle. He admitted he did, so we urged him to relax and open his throat simultaneously with blowing the whistle. He then came forth with an *ah.* We explained that he was pushing some of the air backward into the throat. He soon was able to produce the *ah* at will after blowing the whistle.

Next, we told him to go through the motions of whistling with his lips, but to keep his lips closed, and to feel for air moving backward. That was successful. Shortly, he was able to count from one to ten and to say some of the long vowels. He did not return for further lessons.

One month later. He returned for a medical checkup. The surgeon sent him to the speech clinician. He was speaking fluently with esophageal speech. We admit this was perhaps an unusual demonstration, and there is a probability that he would have been able to use the usual pumping technique, but we wanted to see what we could do with the whistle.

Case 5. Female, age 55. Secretary in a legal office. Patient had had hoarseness off and on for three years, but was given usual medications. Finally, a biopsy was taken after medication would not relieve the hoarseness as it had in the past. Cancer was found on the left vocal fold. Treatment was five weeks of x-ray therapy. No apparent return of the cancer was observed for one year. However, the patient had frequent infections during five years and was treated successfully with antibiotics. Finally, six years after the x-ray treatment, the hoarseness still had not cleared up. A biopsy showed a return on the same vocal fold. One vocal fold was removed by laryngeal fissure. Patient reported the operation was more painful than a later total laryngectomy. At a follow-up examination, cancer was observed on the laryngeal cartilage. Patient delayed surgery for five months. Total laryngectomy finally done. Recovery was good; returned home on the twelfth postoperative day.

Two weeks later. The patient appeared for her first voice lesson. The immediate goal was to demonstrate compression. Used the small plastic whistle to demonstrate moving air backward. Also had the patient puff up cheeks and feel the air move backward as the clinician pressed in the cheeks. She produced an *ah* after using the whistle, then did likewise on a simulated whistle with lips closed. She was asked what was happening to the tongue. She reported that she was pushing it up against the hard palate as she compressed with the lips. With several attempts, she finally produced some esophageal sounds. With a repetition of unvoiced *pah* four times, she followed with a voiced *pah*. She next produced *bah* after compressing with the lips.

Assignments for home practice: experiment with different ways of getting air into the throat. Blow the whistle and when you feel air going down, say *ah*. Inhale with mouth open and say *ah*. Start with a hiss or say *ssss*, followed by /t/; compress with tongue and say *stop*. With lips together, compress them, push tongue up against hard palate and say *ah*. Rapidly say *bah* five times and without voice; then say *bah* with voice. Do it hundreds of times. If successful, try to say *bay, bee, buy, boe, boo* many times. Caution: don't try too hard; stay relaxed. Remember, the sound is made inside the mouth by the lips and tongue, so strain is not necessary.

One week later. Patient able to produce loud sounds of *bah*. Noticed that the patient hesitated after being commanded to say a sound. She indicated she was trying to get organized before saying it. Explained that it takes only an effort to squeeze the air in the mouth back into the throat. Hence, don't wait to get set, just compress and say *pah*. Do it fast in and fast out; it takes only half a second to compress air. To prove that compression was done by tongue, had her bite a knuckle of her finger while compressing air and injecting. She did this well and came forth with a *nah*.

One week later. Patient came in displaying great self-confidence. Immediately said on command: *stop it, get it, take time*, etc. She was doing a slow injection so worked on speed. Used /p/ and /t/ and /k/ said rapidly. Soon she was saying *cup of coffee, O.K., cup of cocoa, skip it*, etc. The patient could not do initial vowels, so used the glide from *pah* to *ah*, followed by *ah* again. Also used *pea-ea, eat*. She quickly mastered these. Assigned words beginning with vowels as well as with plosives.

One week later. Patient seemed to hesitate to inject, although she had talked fluently about her work before the lesson. We explained that she can always start talking merely by saying *pah* or thinking of saying it. "When you are scared, compress your lips and start talking." She at once began to say expressions, like *How are you? Where are you?* and *How do you do?* We next gave her some sentences of six and seven words, expecting her to inject several times. Something unusual happened. The words flowed out at the speed and ease of a normal speaker. The only sign of compression was a slight movement of the lips (see Moolenaar-Bijl). She had caught on to the use of the plosives and intraphrase injection (per Diedrich and Youngstrom), or should we say that she unconsciously used the plosives that way? Henceforth, she had very little problem in fluency.

We obtained lists of words and phrases that she used in her business and dictated them to her. She was urged to practice these at home. This was the last lesson before the teacher left for a convention. We gave her the following instructions:

1. You can say anything now.
2. Take your time; don't be afraid to pause for syllables. Stay relaxed.
3. Say the vowel in every syllable and the last sound of every word.
4. Don't worry about loudness; it will come; get the mechanics first.
5. Remember: you can always start talking if you think of saying *pah-pah*.

Seven weeks later. We telephoned the patient to see if she wished to have a lesson. A woman answered the telephone with a clear, firm voice. She identified herself and said she had taken over the telephone desk and had had no trouble, after her last lesson. She had no problem in being misunderstood. Four years later, she reports her voice is stronger.

Case 6. Male, office manager, age 62 years. He had a history of excessive use of tobacco. Symptom of hoarseness of five weeks' duration. He had never had symptoms like this before. His voice was quite tired after a day of talking over the telephone. He also had smoker's cough which was nonproductive. Biopsy: carcinoma on the left vocal fold with invasion into the muscles of larynx.

Film was shown to patient by speech clinician. Materials given to him to read. Esophageal speech was demonstrated. He also had been told to watch carefully the speech of the laryngectomized persons in the film.

4.17. Total laryngectomy done on left side.

4.30. Patient had healed so rapidly and was in such good physical condition that the laryngologist sent him to the speech clinician on the day of discharge. The patient was in good health and had a wholesome attitude towards his problem. Methods of air intake were demonstrated. He spontaneously injected air and said *bah* and *pah*. He was told to practice saying these two sounds many times until he returned for a second lesson.

Two days later. Patient was able to say *pah, bah and mah* at will and with different vowels.

Two days later. Patient was able to say all vowels; said *Hi* and *OK* and counted from one to five. His voice was high-pitched and quacky.

One day later. Patient had acquired two methods of injecting. He closed his lips when he spoke vowels that began a word, and used the tongue injection for consonants. He was able to say *go* and *gay* without closing his lips. Cooperation was excellent.

Two days later. Patient counted to 100, injecting for each number. He spoke a thirteen-syllable sentence, injecting for each syllable. The pitch of the voice was slightly lower but still quacky and resembling the pharyngeal type. Had him swallow air deliberately to get the feeling for esophageal injection. This helped him to lower his voice slightly: however, he could drawl out diphthongs and was able to say five syllables on one injection.

The patient was anxious to return to work. Since he was now able to communicate with some intelligibility and fluency, the surgeon approved his return. The speech clinician advised him to request an amplified microphone for his telephone in order to increase the loudness of his thin voice. The company approved this and had it installed.

One week later. The patient was able to read all sentences in Waldrop and Gould. He had an occasional loud belch as he read which indicated that air was entering the esophagus. He could talk fluently for a sentence or two and then a gurgling sound was heard. He was told to swallow the saliva, after which the gurgle ceased. He tended to strain while talking and loudness dwindled at the end of sentences. After practicing on taking in a short, quick sniff, he found that he did not have to work so hard at phonating. His chief problem was a short clipping of the vowels and inaccuracy of final consonants. Practice was devoted to prolonging vowels, drawing them out and exaggerating consonants. He was requested to count from twenty to one hundred and to exaggerate every consonant with his lips and teeth. He was urged to do this every morning while he was dressing and to do it in the car as he waited for a red light to turn green.

Two months later. His voice was lower in pitch; the quacky quality had diminished. He still needed practice in articulating /k/ and /g/ and in producing the final consonants of words. Pausing at logical points to take in a breath was practiced.

One month later. The patient was very enthusiastic over having overcome his speech loss. He had resumed all of the duties that he had before at his office. His vowels and consonants were now much more distinct.

Within a year he was doing public speaking for the American Cancer Society to public school children. He recruited a female laryngectomee and two other men to act as a foursome in talking before service clubs and schools. In one month, they talked before 4,000 people. He later became president and a member of the board of directors of a Lost Chord Club. He has reached the eighth postoperative year and has been found to be clear of cancer.

Case 7. A male, barber, age 51 years. He complained of hoarseness over a period of six months. The local physician had treated him for sinusitis. After the hoarseness failed to clear up, the physician took a biopsy and found cancer on the vocal folds.

10.31. The speech clinician was requested to show the film *New Voices* prior to surgery, which was performed by a laryngologist. The patient was given a demonstration of esophageal speech and was told that he would be able to talk one way or another, either by esophageal speech or by an artificial larynx.

11.1 Surgery consisted of right radical neck dissection and removal of portions of the thyroid and parathyroid. Much plastic surgery was done. Slow healing kept the patient in the hospital over one month. The feeding tube was removed on November 30 and he was discharged on December 3. The laboratory report showed that only one node of a chain of seventeen was positive for cancer.

12.17. The patient returned for first postoperative checkup and then was referred to the speech clinician. The patient explained that he had carefully read the material given to him, and that on the way home he had said some words to his wife. He felt that he talked well enough not to have to return for speech work. The speech clinician thought otherwise, but since the patient was in a distant city, he decided he could get along without more therapy.

Eleven years later. The patient coughed up yellow sputum; tired easily. Diagnosis; carcinoma of the right lung. Neck was free of masses and nodes.

Case 8. Male, salesman, age 52 years. The patient entered a clinic because he had a urinary problem. During a complete physical examination, a hard mass was found in the neck at the angle of the jaw (at about the area of the middle one-third of the left anterior lymphatic chain). At biopsy, a frozen section revealed a squamous cell carcinoma, Grade III, on the left aryepiglottic fold and on the false vocal fold. The patient was surprised at this finding, because he thought the discomfort was the result of a tooth extraction some months before.

5.9. Patient was seen by speech clinician who showed the film and demonstrated esophageal voice. It was explained that the possibility for speech was good, either by an artificial larynx or by esophageal speech. A left radical and total larngectomy was performed. The patient was visited daily after returning from the recovery room.

5.23. The patient was discharged with tracheal tube in place; arrangements made for a suction machine. Patient was in excellent health and had a high level of morale.

6.12. The patient returned for a postoperative checkup, and was referred for speech therapy. Demonstrations of different methods of initiating the esophageal sound were given. The patient was able to inject shortly, after several attempts. Later, he was able to inject and produce esophageal sound at will; he then counted up to ten, using one injection for each digit. Within the hour, the patient was able to sustain the voice for two syllables. He advanced so fast that a list of sentences was assigned him. The patient felt so confident that he was able to talk that he did not return for further therapy.

7.19. The patient was referred again to the therapist after a medical checkup proved negative. He used many colloquialisms and could say six syllables on one air-charge. His injection was noisy and resembled a loud swallow. He was urged to relax just before charging air, and to make a slight air intake by sniffing through his nose. This helped him to reduce the loudness of the air-charge. The patient did not return until three months later.

10.9. The laryngologist found a nodule on the right side in the cervical nodular chain. A right radical neck dissection was done. The patient was discharged on October 20.

The following spring, the patient ran for election as a county officer. He traveled 1,000 miles, visiting five towns. He actually entered 5,000 homes to demonstrate that he could talk well and could handle the job. He won with a high majority. When last seen, his speech was fluent; his voice was adequate for a small crowd. On the twelfth postoperative year, he was still free of cancer.

Case 9. Male, farmer, 67 years old. The patient had a history of hoarseness of two months' duration with a more recent loss of phonation and a recurrent bout of dysphagia. A biopsy, laryngeal examination and physical checkup revealed a squamous cell carcinoma that involved 85 per cent of the epiglottis, and had extended to the false vocal folds and to the commissure. The patient was shown the motion picture story *New Voices*, and was coached on injection of air by the 'modified' swallow. He was able to perform this before surgery on the following day.

The patient made a remarkable early recovery from the surgery, a total laryngectomy, and on the seventh post-operative day was discharged. Before he left the hospital, he was sent to the speech clinician for speech instruction. After demonstration of the injection of air, he was able to inject and say *ah* and *bah*. Within a half-hour he said vowels and some short phrases, such as *How are you?*, *Fine* and *Thank you*. He was urged to remain two days before he left for home in a neighboring state. During this time, he acquired the ability to say two-syllable words. Being persuaded to stay two more days, he responded by learning to say short phrases. However, they were indistinct and hastily produced. He was told that he should not hurry; he should take his time rather than slurring his words. In fact, he talked faster than he could swallow air; hence, he whispered and skipped some entire words. We proved to him that he would talk much better if he did not worry about getting the words out. Under these conditions, his speech was more intelligible.

Two weeks later. The patient was whispering and was very upset because he had not learned to talk. Practice was made to use a slow, deliberate type of speech, drawing out the vowels, inhaling frequently and not worrying about getting the words out. Although he demonstrated ability to do this, he still displayed anxiety about not talking.

Five weeks later, he returned in a great state of anxiety. He insisted that he had to have an artificial larynx because he could not talk to his wife, who was ill. Also, he said that his dog just wagged his tail when he asked him to go get the cows. The patient was given the name of an agent near him, but was urged to keep on trying.

Six months later. The patient returned for a medical checkup. He was calm and contented, and using adequate esophageal speech. He had purchased the instrument but later found that he was able to talk with esophageal speech. A good question here is whether the instrument gave him the confidence of being able to communicate, and whether the acquired skill necessary for articulating with an instrument had given him the skill that was also necessary for using esophageal speech.

Case 10. Male, 43 years old, poultry worker, weighing over 225 pounds. Biopsy produced a squamous cell cancer on the right vocal fold which extended beyond the commissure to the left vocal fold. The patient and his wife were shown the film *New Voices,* and also methods of injecting air. He had been a beer drinker and was able to eruct on command. On the third day after surgery, he was up and walking around, carrying the feeding tube with him. He complained that those liquids were not enough food; he was starving. Because of quick recovery, he was started on speech lessons on the eleventh postoperative day. He could belch several times in succession and assured us that he was going to talk. Assignments were to inject air and say the first word list in Waldrop and Gould. Two days later, he spoke these words spontaneously along with some three-word phrases. At the end of an hour, he read a sixteen-word sentence and enthusiastically threw his writing pad to the floor.

Five days later. The patient was using three- and four-syllable words but complained about stomach disorders. He was trained to take small air-charges in an easy relaxed manner. Six weeks after surgery, he was cleared for return to work.

Case 11. An eighty-year-old man had a simple laryngectomy. Although he was shown the film *New Voices,* and was given a demonstration of esophageal speech, he was not interested in learning to talk. He had brought his sons with him to see the film. They, likewise, were not interested in their father learning to use esophageal speech. After the father recovered and was ready to leave the hospital, they asked for the name of a salesman who could sell them an artificial larynx for their father.

Case 12. A sixty-year-old male factory worker had simple laryngectomy. Six days after surgery, the patient was affected by violent gastric disturbances. It was revealed that he had been a heavy drinker and had acquired a gastric ulcer. This had been reactivated by frequent entrance of air into his stomach He was kept in the hospital for six weeks before the ulcer was healed. In order to forestall any recurrence of the attack, the surgeon instructed the speech clinician to advise the patient to obtain an artificial larynx.

Case 13. Bar tender, 57 years old, had chronic laryngitis in 1949. He was advised to stop all tobacco. He continued to smoke forty cigarettes a day and his hoarseness continued. Although he had said that he was a moderate drinker, he admitted taking three jiggers of whisky daily.

12.8.60. The patient came in because he had a pain in the area of the angle of the jaw. He had had mumps eighteen months before and thought this was an aftereffect. Complained of difficulty in swallowing; that the pain recurred whenever he talked or sneezed.

First impression was hypertrophic granular tissue on the left false vocal fold. The right false vocal fold appeared to be normal. Biopsy found cancer, squamous cell Grade III.

1.15.61. Motion picture *New Voices* shown. Patient was instructed to watch the lips of the actors to see how they talked without vocal cords.

1.16.61. Laryngectomy and hemithyroidectomy.

2.2.61. First speech lesson. Worked on injection. Since he had been a drinker, he was able to belch well; in fact, too well. Five minutes after the demonstration of injection, he spoke twenty-five words. Assigned first word list in Waldrop and Gould.

2.16.61. Speech was not as good as expected. He was using a full swallow, and belch was forceful. Emphasized tongue compression rather than swallow, with a quick injection and quick return.

2.23.61. Patient was able to make injections every three seconds. Practice was directed toward prolonging vowels, and saying familiar words used at the bar, such as *Hi, OK, Yes, No,* etc. Had him walk around, swinging arms as he talked. The relaxation tended to give him more fluent speech and reduced the habit of making a loud belch.

3.13.61. Came in saying two and three vowels on one expulsion. He reported that he could talk to his wife, who could understand him.

4.6.61. Patient returned with too long a belch, which slowed up fluency. He admitted that he had not done well, so he had begun to drink too much of his own merchandise. He resorted to the whistle technique and got four good expulsions on one injection. Assigned quick in-and-out action.

4.13.61. Patient was using better compression and abdominal press. Was able to say *bah* four times on one expulsion and counted to ten with ease. Worked on rapid injection and return to reduce excessive air expulsion.

4.30.61. Patient made ten straight injections and expulsions, and demonstrated increased vocabulary. The lag between injection and expulsion was chief problem. Worked on tongue injection and quick expulsion.

5.15.61. Was able to talk with three syllables per air-charge. Was told to relax and talk without excessive tension around neck and face.

6.8.61. Patient was speaking three-syllable words. Counted to seven on one injection. Worked on prolonging vowels, consonants and sentences. Patient did not return.

11.12.69. Still tending bar.

Case 14. This case is an example of poor communication or failure of the clinician to realize that the patient had not understood instructions. The patient thought that the air had to go on into the stomach before he could use it. This caused much delay and confusion.

Barber, 63 years old. Complained of hoarseness for eight years, especially after excessive talking. In the spring of 1958, he lost his voice but did nothing about it. In August, laryngologist's impression was hyperkeratosis.

10.28.58. Biopsy found cancer. Motion picture shown; pamphlets given.

11.3.58. Radical neck on left side and total laryngectomy; also hemithyroidectomy. Fistula developed which kept patient in hospital a month.

12.8.58. First speech lesson. Patient appeared to be intelligent and cooperative, but was very nervous and tense, to the extent that there was no success in getting injection.

12.17.58. Patient still tense; was losing his business because people were afraid of cancer and he could not talk. (We never thought of an artificial larynx!)

12.31.58. Still too tense. Patient reported that he could only swallow tiny pieces of meat; the fistula probably had caused a narrowing of the esophagus. Patient did not return. Admitted he was unable to pay for therapy.

4.1.59. Clinician obtained sponsor for the patient. Patient urged to come back. He indicated that he had the wrong idea. He thought he had to swallow air into the stomach. He was complaining of gastric distress. We worked on quick expulsion. Got the idea of pumping air down with tongue.

4.15.59. Patient still having difficulty expelling air. Trained him to sniff a bit of air before injecting. He at once got *bah* and then was able to say nine straight syllables of *bah*.

4.22.59. Counted to ten; able to do phrases and short sentences.

4.29.59. Worked on phrases and sentences. Patient very encouraged. Used a nine-word sentence, urging him to pronounce every vowel distinctly.

6.9.59. Patient had had a fall and broke several ribs. Being bandaged, he was unable to get in enough air and voice was soft. This was a demonstration of importance of thoracic and diaphragmatic action. When he was encouraged to use the lower ribs and the expansion of the substernal abdomen, he got better support for voice. This appeared to help him to establish fluency and continuity.

12.13.61. Cancer found under the thyroid lobe. The eight years of hoarseness without medical attention had finally brought its toll.

Case 15. Male, age 51. Polisher in factory. Had sore throat for six months. Pain was referred to the right ear. Voice was hoarse. Patient had smoked 1½ packages of cigarettes daily since he was fifteen years old. Throat was full of mucus.

Examination: right side of larynx edematous; right vocal cord fixed; neoplastic mass extended to false vocal cord. Fullness up to the vallecula.

4.16.63. Total laryngectomy.

4.30.63. Patient seen on day of discharge, he wanted to talk; said *bah* easily. Clinician warned him not to try it until he returned for first lesson.

5.14.63. Patient was able to say two- and three-syllable words by injection. Also said five and six words in a sentence.

5.28.63. Patient was able to read the Gettysburg Address. Showed facial grimaces. Used mirror to correct these. Patient wanted to return to work.

6.13.63. Fellow workmen called him "Blabbermouth." Since he was a polisher, he asked for a mask. The surgeon wrote letter to factory to recommend that a mask be used. The patient was furnished one.

7.1.63. The patient's diadokinesis was as rapid as a normal person's. He bragged that he had never used a pencil and pad from the beginning.

2.19.69. The patient was still working and clear of cancer.

REFERENCES

Anderson, J.O. (1950): A descriptive study of elements of esophageal speech. Unpublished Ph.D. dissertation, Ohio State University, Columbus.

Anderson, V. (1961): *Training the Speaking Voice*. New York, Oxford.

Andrews, A.H., Jr. (1957): Panel on visitation. Convention of International Association of Laryngectomees, Milwaukee, Wisc., August 15, 1957.

Arnold, G.E. (1960): Alleviation of alaryngeal aphonia with the modern artificial larynx. I. Evolution of artificial speech aids and their value for rehabilitation. *Logos*, 3:55–67.

Baker, G.L. (1965): Correspondence (See Lauder 1965).

Bangs, J.L.; Lierle, D.M., and Strother, C.R. (1946): Speech after laryngectomy. *J Speech Dis*, 11:171–76.

Barney, H.L. (1958): A discussion of some technical aspects of speech aids for post-laryngectomized patients. *Ann Otol (St Louis)*, 67:1–13.

Barton, J., and Hejna, R. (1963): Factors associated with success or nonsuccess in acquisition of esophageal speech. *J Speech Hearing Ass (Virginia)*, 4:19–20.

Bateman, G.H. (1953): Oesophageal speech after laryngectomy. *Acta Otolaryng (Stockholm)*, 43:133–39.

Bateman, G.H., and Negus, V.E. (1954): Speech after laryngectomy. *Brit Surg Progr*, p. 105.

Bateman, G.H.; Dornhorst, A., and Leathhart, G. (1952): Oesophageal speech. *Brit Med J*, 2:1177–78.

Beck, J. (1954): Phonetische Untersuchungen an Laryngektomierten (Phonetic examinations in laryngectomized). *Arch Ohr Nas Kehlkopfheilk*, 165:576–81.

Behringer, S.M. (1965): Correspondence (See Lauder 1965).

Berg, J. van den, and Moolenaar Bijl, A.J. (1959): Cricopharyngeal sphincter, pitch, intensity and fluency in oesophageal speech. *Prac Otorhinolaryng (Basel)*, 21:298–315.

Berg, J. van den; Moolenaar-Biji, A.J., and Damsté, P.H. (1958): Oesophageal speech. *Folia Phonat (Basel)*, 10:65–84.

Berlin, C.I. (1963a): Clinical measurement of esophageal speech. I. Methodology and curves of skill acquisition. *J Speech Hearing Dis*, 28:42–51.

Berlin, C.I. (1963b): Clinical measurement of esophageal speech. II. An unexpected dividend. *J Speech Hearing Dis*, 28:398–92.

Berlin, C.I. (1964): Hearing loss, palatal function and other factors in postlaryngectomy rehabilitation. *J Chronic Dis*, 17:677–84.

Berlin, C.I. (1965a): Clinical measurement of esophageal speech. III. Performance of non-biased groups. *J Speech Hearing Dis*, 30:174–83.

Berlin, C.I. (1965b): Correspondence (See Lauder 1965).

Berry, M.E., and Eisenson, J. (1956): *Speech Disorders. Principles and Practices of Therapy*. New York. Appleton.

Bisi, R.H., and Conley, J.J. (1965): Psychologic factors influencing vocal rehabilitation of the post-laryngectomy patient. *Ann Otol*, 74:1073–78.

Bondarenko, E.D. (1962): Rasvitie Zvuchnoi rechi u bol'nykh posle laringektomii (Development of voiced speech in patients after laryngectomy). *Vestn Otorinolaring*, 24:77–79.

Brighton, G.R., and Boone, W.H. (1937): Roentgenographic demonstration of method of speech in cases of complete laryngectomy. *Amer J Roentgen*, 38:571–83.

Brodnitz, F.S. (1959): *Vocal Rehabilitation*. Rochester, Whiting.

Chen, L.-C.Y.; Samberg, H.M., and Felsenstein, B. (1963): Aspects of rehabilitation of the laryngectomized patient. *Arch Phys Med Rehab, 44:*267–72.

Clark, A.F. (1965): Correspondence (See Lauder 1965).

Cojazzi, L. (1949): Sulla funzione esofagea fonetica vicario vicariante nei laringecto-mizzatti. *Atti Laborat Fonetica Univ Padua, 1:*41.

Conley, J.J.; Deamesti, F., and Pierce, M.K. (1958): A new surgical technique for the vocal rehabilitation of the laryngectomized patient. *Ann Otol, 67:*655–64.

Corgill, D.A. (1965): Correspondence (See Lauder 1965).

Crouse, G.P. (1962): An experimental study of esophageal and artificial speech. Unpublished Master's thesis, Emory University, Atlanta, Ga.

Curran, V. (1965): Correspondence (See Lauder 1965).

Czermak, J. (1859): Uber die Sprache bei luftdichter Verschliessung des Kehlkopfs. *S B Acad Wiss Wien, 35:*65.

Damsté, P.H. (1958): *Oesophageal Speech After Laryngectomy*. Groningen, Gebr. Hortsema.

Damsté, P.H. (1959): Glosso-pharyngeal press. *Speech Path Ther, 2:*70–76.

Damsté, P.H.; Berg, J. van den, and Moolenaar-Bijl, A.J. (1956): Why are some patients unable to learn esophageal speech? *Ann Otol, 65:*998–1005.

Darley, F.L. (1963): Special problems in aging. *Postgrad Med, 33:*294–300.

Darley, F.L. (1964): *Diagnosis and Appraisal of Communication Disorders*. Englewood Cliffs, N.J., Prentice-Hall.

Decroix, G.; Libersa, C., and Lattard, R. (1958): Bases anatomiques et physiologiques de la rééducation vocale des laryngectomises (The anatomical and physiological foundation of voice reeducation in laryngectomees). *J Franc Otolaryng, 7:*549–73.

DiCarlo, L.M.; Amster, W., and Herer, G. (1955): *Speech After Laryngectomy*. Syracuse, Syracuse.

Diedrich, W.M., and Youngstrom, K. (1966): *Alaryngeal Speech*. Springfield, Thomas.

Doehler, M.E. (1953): *Esophageal Speech*. Boston, American Cancer Society.

Ehrlich, N. (1937): *The Life of a Laryngectomee*. New York, Froben.

Equen, M. (1956): The rehabilitation of the laryngectomee. *Arch Otolaryng (Chicago), 64:*1–2.

Equen, M. (1965): Correspondence (See Lauder 1965).

Ferguson, J.D. (1965): Correspondence (See Lauder 1965).

Finkbeiner, E.R. (1968): Surgery and speech, the pseudoglottis, and respiration in total standard laryngectomy. (In Snidecor 1968).

Fletcher, H. (1953): *Speech and Hearing in Communication*. New York, Van Nostrand.

Fontaine, A., and Mitchell, J. (1960): Oesophageal voice; a factor of readiness. *J Laryng, 74:*870–76.

Frankel, B. (1893): Ueuber den kunstlichen Kehlkopf und die Pseudostimme. *Berl Klin Wschr, 31:*756.

Freud, E.D. (1948): Speech therapy: experience with patients who had undergone total laryngectomy. *Arch Otolaryng (Chicago), 48:*150–55.

Froeschels, E. (1951): Therapy of the alaryngeal voice following laryngectomy; a contribution. *Arch Otolaryng (Chicago), 53:*77–62.

Gardner, W.H. (1951): Rehabilitation after laryngectomy. *Public Health Nurs (New York, 43:*612–15.

Gardner, W.H. (1954): They will talk again. *Nurs Outlook, 2:*314–15, 1954.

Gardner, W.H. (1956): Report on gastric disorders of laryngectomized persons. Convention of International Association of Laryngettomees, Miami, Fla., 1956.

Gardner, W.H. (1961): Problems of laryngectomees. *J Chronic Dis, 13*:253–60.

Gardner, W.H. (1962a): The whistle technique in esophageal speech. *J Speech Hearing Dis, 27*:187–88.

Gardner, W.H. (1962b): Tenth anniversary history of IAL. Convention of International Association of Laryngectomees, Memphis, Tenn., August 21, 1962.

Gardner, W.H. (1964): Laryngectomees (neck breathers) in industry. *Arch Environ Health (Chicago), 9*:777–89.

Gardner, W.H. (1966): Adjustment problems of laryngectomized women. *Arch Otolaryng (Chicago), 83*:31–42.

Gardner, W.H., and Harris, H.E. (1961): Aids and devices for laryngectomees. *Arch Otolaryng (Chicago), 73*:145–52.

Gatewood, E.T. (1945): A simple and practical procedure for developing esophageal voice in the laryngectomized patient. *Ann Otol, 54*:322–27.

Genereaux, K.S. (1968): Correspondence (Quoted in Snidecor 1968).

Gilmore, S.L. (1961): Rehabilitation after laryngectomy. *Amer J Nurs, 61*:87–89.

Gilse, P.H.G. van (1949): Another method of speech without larynx. *Acta Otolaryng (Stockholm), 78*:109–10.

Greene, J.S. (1947): Laryngectomy and its psychological implications. *New York J Med, 47*:53–56.

Greene, M.C.L. (1964): *The Voice and Its Disorders,* 2nd ed. Philadelphia, Lippincott.

Gussenbauer, C. (1874): Uber die erste druch Th. Billroth am Menschen ausgefuehrte Kehlkopf-Exstirpation under die Anwendung eines Kuenstlichen Kehlkopfes. *Arch Klin Chir, 17*:343–56.

Gutzmann, H., Sr. (1909): Stimme und sprache ohne kehlkopf. *Z Laryng Rhinol Otol, 1*:221.

Haase, H.J. (1960): Psychologie under Psychopathologie Kehlkopfexstirpierter. Zur Bedeutungvon Personlichkeitsanlage, Erlebnis und Milieu (Psychology and psychopathology after laryngectomy). *Fortschr Neurol Psychiat, 28*:253–72.

Hahn, E.; Lomas, C.W.; Hargis, D.E., and Vandraegan, D. (1957): *Basic Voice Training for Speech.* New York, McGraw-Hill.

Hanley, T.D., and Thurman, W.L. (1962): *Developing Vocal Skills.* New York, Holt, Rinehart & Winston.

Harrington, R. (1960): Problems associated with the development of pseudo-voice in the aged laryngectomee. Convention Report, American Speech and Hearing Association, Los Angeles, Nov. 1960.

Heaver, L., and Arnold, G.E. (1962): Rehabilitation of alaryngeal aphonia. *Postgrad Med, 32*:11–17.

Heaver, L.; White, W., and Goldstein, N. (1955): Clinical experience in restoring oral communication to 274 laryngectomized patients by esophageal voice. *J Amer Geriat Soc, 3*:687–90.

Hodson, C.J., and Oswald, M.V.O. (1958): *Speech Recovery after Total Laryngectomy.* Baltimore, Williams and Wilkins.

Holinger, P.H.; Johnston, K.C., and Mansueto, M.D. (1957): Cancer of the larynx. I. Surgical treatment *Amer J Nurs, 57*:738–41.

Hollyfield, M. (1965): Correspondence (See Lauder 1965).

Horn, D. (1962): Summary: Laryngectomee survey report. Convention of International Association of Laryngectomees, Memphis, Tenn., August 21, 1962.

Howie, T.O. (1946): Rehabilitation after total laryngectomy: Successful esophageal speech. *Glasg Med J*, 27:45–48.

Huber, N.W., and Kopp, G.A. (1942): *The Practice of Speech Correction in the Medical Clinic.* Boston, Expression Company.

Hyman, M. (1955): An experimental study of artificial larynx and esophageal speech. *J Speech Hearing Dis*, 20:291–99.

Hyman, M. (1960): *How To Speak Again* (a manual with a recording of instructions for laryngectomees). Cleveland, American Cancer Society.

Hyman, M. (1965): Correspondence (See Lauder 1965).

International Association of Laryngectomees, *Directory*. New York, IAL (published annually).

Irwin, J.A. (1964): Report: Clubs' services to laryngectomees. Convention of International Association of Laryngectomees, New York, August, 1964.

Isshiki, N., and Snidecor, J.C. (1965): Air intake and usage in esophageal speech. *Acta Otolaryng (Stockholm)*, 59:559–74.

Jackson, C.L. (1940): The voice after direct laryngoscopic operations, laryngofissure and laryngectomy. *Arch Otolaryng (Chicago)*, 31:23–37.

Janowski, W.; Kaniowski, T., and Reczek, H.L. (1959): Radidlogickzen obrazy gardla dolego u beskrtaniowcow (The x-ray picture of the hypopharynx in laryngectomized patients). *Pol Przegl Radjol*, 23:15–18.

Jesberg, N. (1954): Rehabilitation after laryngectomy. *Calif Med*, 80:80–82.

Jimison, C. (1957): Cancer of the larynx. II. Nursing the patient after laryngectomy. *Amer J Nurs*, 57:741–43.

Johannessen, J.V., and Foy, A.L. (1964): Team effort in the rehabilitation of laryngectomy patients. *J Amer Geriat Soc.* 12:1073–76.

Johnson, C.L. (1960): A survey of laryngectomee patients in Veteran's Administration hospitals. *Arch Otolaryng (Chicago)*, 72:768–73.

Judson, L.S., and Weaver, A.T. (1942): *Voice Science.* New York, Crofts.

Kallen, L.A. (1934): Vicarious vocal mechanisms: The anatomy, physiology and development of speech in laryngectomized persons. *Arch Otolaryng (Chicago)*, 20: 460–503.

Keenan, J.P. (1965): Correspondence (See Lauder 1965).

Kindler, W. (1960): Die Rehabilitation Kehlkopfloser nach Krebsausrottung (Rehabilitation of laryngectomees after extirpation of cancer) *Med Welt*, 35:1748–50.

Klieger, P.A. (1966): Background material on cancer research and rehabilitation. *A Conference on Research Needs in the Rehabilitation of Persons with Disabilities Resulting from Cancer.* New York, VRA and Institute of Physical Medicine and Rehabilitation. N.Y.U. Medical Center, 1966, pp. 55–71.

Knepflar, K.J. (1960): Individualized speech therapy for laryngectomized patients. Convention Report. American Speech and Hearing Association, Los Angeles, 1960.

Knox, A.W. (1965): Correspondence (See Lauder 1965).

Kusske, B.W. (1957): Panel: Visitation to laryngectomized patients. Convention of International Association of Laryngectomees, St. Paul, Minn., August 1957.

Laguaite, J.K. (1962): Psychological and social problems of the laryngectomized individual. *Short Course on Esophageal Speech.* New York, American Speech and Hearing Association.

Laguaite, J.K., and Waldrop, W.F. (1963): Acoustic analysis of fundamental frequency of voice before and after therapy. *N Z Speech Therapist J*, 18:23–25.

Lanpher, A. (1965a): Correspondence (See Lauder 1965).

Lanpher, A. (1965b): Hello Tallulah. In Ross, W., *The Climate Is Hope*. Englewood Cliffs, N.J., Prentice-Hall.

Lanpher, A. (1967): Making the voice feminine. *IAL News*, December 1967.

Lauder, E.M. (1965): The role of the laryngectomee in post-laryngectomy voice instruction. *J Speech Hearing Dis* 30:145–58.

Lauder, E.M. (1968): *Self-Help for the Laryngectomee*. 6334 Dove Hill Dr., San Antonio, Tex. 78238.

Levin, N.M. (1940): Teaching the laryngectomized patient to talk. *Arch Otolaryng (Chicago)*, 32:299–314.

Levin, N.M. (1952): Speech rehabilitation after total removal of larynx. *JAMA, 149:* 1281–86.

Levin, N.M. (1955): Total laryngectomy and speech rehabilitation. *Eye Ear Nose Throat Monthly, 34:*585–92.

Levin, N.M. (Ed.) (1962): *Voice and Speech Disorders: Medical Aspects* Springfield, Thomas.

Levin, N.M. (1965): Correspondence (See Lauder 1965).

Lindsay, J.R.; Morgan, R.H., and Wepman, J.M. (1954): The cricopharyngeus muscle in esophageal speech *Laryngoscope, 54:*55–65.

Locke, B. (1966): Psychology of the laryngectomee. *Military Medicine*, July 1966, pp. 593–99.

Loebell, H., and Brahm, K. (1950): Gibt es beim Normalen einem Glottis-bzw. Sphinkterverschluss beim Heben von leichteren Gewichten (20 Kg.) und wie stent der Kehlkopftotalestirpierte den alltaglichen Balastungen gegenuber? *Folia Phoniat (Basel)*, 2:67–68.

Long, P.H. (1960): On being a laryngectomee. *Medical Times*, December 1960.

Luchsinger, R., and Arnold, G.E. (1965): *Voice-Speech-Language. Clinical Communicology: Its Physiology and Pathology*. Belmont, Calif., Wadsworth.

Malbeck, E., and Schlosshauer, B. (1960): Phonatrische nach untersuchungen chordecktomierter patienten (Phoniatric examinations of Cordectomized patients). *HNO*, 8:201–205.

Marge, M. (1965): Tongue thrust and alaryngeal voice training. *J Speech Hearing Dis*, 30:376–77.

Marland, P.M. (1949): A direct method of teaching voice after total laryngectomy. *Speech, 13:*4–13.

Martin, H. (1950): Esophageal speech. *Ann Otol*, 59:687–89.

Martin, H. (1955): Speech rehabilitation following laryngectomy; general consideration. *Talk, 36:*4–6.

Martin, H. (1963): Rehabilitation of the laryngectomee. *Cancer, 16:*823–41.

Mawhinney, C.K. (1965): Correspondence (See Lauder 1965).

McCall, J.W. (1943): Preliminary voice training for laryngectomy. *Arch Otolaryng (Chicago)*, 38:10–16.

McCall, J.W. (1953): Improvement of surgical techniques for removal of the larynx. Summary. Second Annual Institute on Voice Pathology. Cleveland Hearing and Speech Center, Cleveland, Ohio, August 10–15, 1953.

McCall, J.W., and Fisher, W.R. (1952): Carcinoma of the larynx. A report of 194 cases with 149 laryngectomees. *Laryngoscope, 62:*475–85.

McCall, J.W., and Stover, W.C. (1944): Laryngectomy for laryngeal cancer: A review of 45 cases. *Laryngoscope, 54:*659–76.

McCall, J.W.; Hendershot, E.L., and Whitaker, C.W. (1960): Cancer of the larynx and epiglottis. *Ohio State Med J, 56:*329–33.

McClear, J. (1959: Report on successful speech in patients with excessive tissue removed. *Anamilo Nat Courier.* New York, National Hospital for Speech Disorders, February 1959.

McClear, J. (1960): *Esophageal Voice Production. An Instruction Manual.* New York, National Hospital for Speech Disorders.

McClear, J. (1969): *Your Second Voice.* New York, Speech Rehabilitation Institute.

McCroskey, R.L., and Mulligan, M. (1963): The relative intelligibility of esophageal speech and artificial larynx speech. *J Speech Hearing Dis, 28:*37–41.

Miller, M.H. (1959): The responsibility of the speech therapy to the laryngectomized patient. *Arch Otolaryng (Chicago),* 70:211–16.

Miller, A.H. (1967): First experiences with the Asai technique for vocal rehabilitation after total laryngectomy. *Ann Otol,* 76:829–33 (See also Chapter 3 in Snidecor 1968.)

Montreuil, F. (1960): Cancer of the larynx. *Canad Med Ass J,* 82:1216–19.

Moolenaar-Bijl, A.J. (1951): Some data on speech without a larynx. *Folia Phoniat (Basel),* 3:1:20–24.

Moolenaar-Bijl, A.J. (1953a): Connection between consonant articulation and the intake of air in oesophageal speech. *Folia Phoniat (Basel),* 5:212–15.

Moolenaar-Bijl, A.J. (1953b): The importance of certain consonants in oesophageal voice after laryngectomy. *Ann Otol,* 62:979.

Moore, G.P. (1953): Discussion. Summary. Second Annual Institute on Voice Pathology. Cleveland Hearing and Speech Center, Cleveland, Ohio, August 10–15, 1953.

Moore, G.P. (1957): Voice disorders associated with organic voice abnormalities. In Travis, L.E. (Ed): *Handbook of Speech Pathology.* New York, Appleton.

Moore, G.P. (1965): Correspondence (See Lauder 1965).

Moore, G.P., and Koepp-Baker, H. (1948): The rehabilitation of the laryngectomized. *Trans Amer Acad Opth Otolaryng,* 52:227.

Morrison, W.W. (1931): The production of voice and speech after total laryngectomy. *Arch Otolaryng (Chicago),* 14:413–23.

Morrison, W.W. (1941): Physical rehabilitation of the laryngectomized patient. *Arch Otolaryng (Chicago),* 34:1101–12.

Moses, P.J. (1958): Rehabilitation of the post-laryngectomized patient; the vocal therapist and contribution to the rehabilitation program. *Ann Otol,* 67:538–43.

Moses, P.J. (1965): Correspondence (See Lauder 1965).

Motta, G.; Profazio, A., and Acciarri, T. (1959): Osservasioni roentgencinematografiche sulla fonzione nei laryngectomizzati (Roentgenocinematographic observations on the phonation of laryngectomized subjects). *Otorinolaryng (Ital),* 28:261–86.

Murphy, A.T. (1964): *Functional Voice Disorders.* Englewood Cliffs, N.J., Prentice-Hall.

Nahum, A.M., and Golden, J.S. (1963): Psychological problems of laryngectomy. *JAMA,* 186:1136–38.

Negus, E. (1938): Affectations of the cricopharyngeal fold. *Laryngoscope,* 48:107–58.

Nelson, C.R. (1949): *Post-laryngectomy Speech. You Can Speak Again.* New York, Funk & Wagnalls.

Nessel, E. (1963): Kunstliche Kehlkopfe (Artificial larynx). *HNO,* 11:249–53.

Nichols, A.C. (1968): Loudness and quality in esophageal speech and the artificial larynx. Chap. VII in Snidecor 1968.

Norris, C.M. (1958): Rehabilitation of the postlaryngectomized patient. 1. Types of clinical cases and their resultant esophageal, pharyngeal and neck deformities. *Ann Otol*, 67:528–37.

Ogura, J.H. (1960): Cancer of the larynx, pharynx and upper cervical esophagus. *Arch Otolaryng (Chicago)*, 72:66–72.

Orton, H.B. (1941): Remarks at American Laryngology Association annual meeting, 1941. *Arch Otolaryng (Chicago)* 34:679–81.

Peacher, G. (1966): *How To Improve Your Speaking Voice*. New York, Frederick Fell.

Pekarek, V.F. (1967): Report: The advantage of being a neck breather. Convention of International Association of Laryngectomees, Chicago, 1966. *IAL News*, April 1967.

Pellegrini, V. (1957): On the so-called pseudo-glottis in laryngectomized persons. *J Laryng*, 71:405–10.

Perello, J. (1951a): El problema de la voz en los laringectomizdos (The problems of the voice in laryngectomized persons). *Acta Otorinolaring (Iber Amer)*, vol. 3.

Perello, J. (1951b): La educación foniátrica de los laringectomizdos (Phoniatric education of laryngectomized persons). *Med Clin (Barcelona)*, 17:251–53.

Perello, J. (1953): La voix du laryngectomizé. *La Voix*, 1:317–34. Paris, Maloine.

Pichler, J.H. (1961): Uber ein neuartiges Autmatisch Gesteuertes Elektronisches Sperechgerat fur Laryngektomierte (On a new automatic controlled electronic speech apparatus for laryngectomees). *Acta otolaryngol*, 53:374–80.

Pitkin, Y. (1953): Factors affecting psychologic adjustment in the laryngectomized patient. *Arch Otolaryng*, 58:38–49.

Pitkin, Y. (1965): Correspondence (See Lauder 1965).

Pond, N.L.: Personal conversation.

Putney, F.J. (1958): Rehabilitation of post-laryngectomized patients. Specific discussion of failures; advanced and difficult technical problems. *Ann Otol*, 67:544–49.

Ranney, J.L. (1965): Report on unemployment of laryngectomees. *IAL News*, 10:1.

Ranney, J.L. (1969): Help for the laryngectomee. *Physician's Management,* June 1969, suppl. pp. 69, 70, 76, 79.

Reed, G.F., and Snow, J.B., Jr. (1960): Reappraisal of seventy-five cases of radical neck dissection for carcinoma of the larynx. *Ann Otol*, 69:271–79.

Rickenberg, H.E. (1953): Laryngectomized speech. *Arch Otolaryng (Chicago)*, 58: 421–24.

Robe, E.Y.; Moore, P.; Andrews, A.H., Jr., and Holinger, P.H. (1956): A study of the role of certain factors in the development of speech after laryngectomy. 1. Type of operation. *Laryngoscope*, 66:173–86, 1956a; 2. Site of pseudoglottis. *Laryngoscope*, 66:382–401, 1956b; 3. Coordination of speech with respiration. *Laryngoscope*, 66:481–99, 1956c.

Ross, L.E. (1965): Correspondence (See Lauder 1965).

Sawkins, J. (1949): Voice without a larynx. *The Medical Press*, 222, No. 5756, August 31, 1949.

Sawkins, J. (1952): Private correspondence.

Schall, L.A. (1938): Psychology of laryngectomized patients. *Arch Otolaryng*, 28: 581–87.

Schall, L.A. (1954): The patient after laryngectomy. In Ellis, M.: *Modern Trends in Diseases of Ear, Nose and Throat*. New York, Hoeber.

Schilling, R., and Binder, R.H. (1927): Uber die Pharnyx- und Oesophagusstimme. *Zbl Ohrenheilk*, 9:893.

Schlosshauer, B., and Möckel, G. (1958): Answertung der Rontgentonfilm aufnahmen von Speiserohrensprechen (Interpretation of roentgen sound films made of esophageal speakers). *Folia Phoniat, 10:*154–66.

Seeman, M. (1958): Zur Pathologie der Osphagusstimme (Pathology of the esophageal voice). *Folia Phoniat (Basel), 10:*44–50.

Seeman, M. (1967): Rehabilitation of laryngectomized subjects. *Acta Otolaryng (Stockholm), 61:*235–41.

Shames, G.H.; Font, J., and Matthews, J. (1963): Factors related to speech proficiency of the laryngectomized. *J Speech Hearing Dis, 28:*273–87.

Shanks, J.C. (1965): Correspondence (See Lauder 1965).

Shanks, J.C. (1967): Advantages in the use of esophageal speech by a laryngectomee. *Laryngoscope, 77:*239–43.

Smith, J.K.; Rise, E.N., and Gralnek, D.E. (1966): Speech recovery in laryngectomized patients. *Laryngoscope, 76:*1540–46.

Snidecor, JC. (1965): Correspondence (See Lauder 1965).

Snidecor, J.C. (1968): *Speech Rehabilitation of the Laryngectomized,* rev. ed. Springfield, Thomas.

Snidecor, J.C., and Curry, E.T. (1959): Temporal and pitch aspects of superior esophageal speech. *Ann Otol. 68:*623–36.

Sparks, B.: Private communication.

Stetson, R.H. (1933): Speech movements in action. *Trans Amer Laryng Ass, 55:*29–42.

Stetson, R.H. (1937a): Esophageal speech for any laryngectomized person. *Arch Otolaryng (Chicago), 26:*132–42.

Stetson, R.H. (1937b): Can all laryngectomized patients be taught esophageal speech? *Trans Amer Laryng Ass, 59:*59–71.

Stoll, B. (1958): Psychological factors determining the success or failure of the rehabilitation program of laryngectomized patients. *Ann Otol, 67:*550–57.

Stoll, B. (1965): Correspondence (See Lauder 1965).

Strother, C. (1948): In Froeschels, E.: *Twentieth Century Speech and Voice Correction.* Philadelphia, Philosophical Library, pp. 302–12.

Svane-Knudson, V. (1960): The substitute voice of the laryngectomized patient. *Acta Otolaryng (Stockholm), 52:*85–93.

Tait, V., and Tait, R.V. (1959): Speech rehabilitation with the oral vibrator. *Speech Path Ther, 2:*64–69.

Taub, S. (1970): A new method of surgery for developing pulmonary air for postlaryngectomy speech. Paper delivered with demonstration of a patient to IAL Convention, Buffalo, N.Y., July 28, 1970.

Tikofsky, R.P.; Glattke, J.J., and Perry, P.S. (1964): Listener identification of esophageal production of voiced consonants. Report: Convention of American Speech and Hearing Association, San Francisco, Calif., 1964.

Van Riper, C. (1963): *Speech Correction, Principles and Methods,* 4th ed. Englewood Cliffs, N.J., Prentice-Hall.

Van Riper, C., and Irwin, J.V. (1958): *Voice and Articulation.* Englewood Cliffs, N.J., Prentice-Hall.

Vrticka, K., and Svoboda, M. (1963): Time changes in the x-ray picture of the hypopharynx, pseudoglottis and in the esophagus in the course of vocal rehabilitation of 70 laryngectomized speakers. *Folia Phoniat, 15:*1–12.

Waldrop, W.F. (1965): Correspondence (See Lauder 1965).

Waldrop, W.F., and Baker, G.L. (1966): Speeding rehabilitation of the laryngectomee. *A Conference on Research Needs in the Rehabilitation of Persons with Disabilities*

Resulting from Cancer. New York, VRA and Institute of Physical Medicine and Rehabilitation. N.Y.U. Medical Center, 1966, pp. 55–71.

Waldrop, W.F., and Gould, M.A. (1956): *Your New Voice.* Chicago, Ill., American Cancer Society.

Waldrop, W.F., and Toht, A.E. (1958): Analyses of vowels of laryngectomized speakers. Report: Convention of American Speech and Hearing Association, New York, 1958.

Weihs, H. (1958): Der ein fluss behachbarter Bewegungsysteme auf die Hervolbringung der Oesophagussprache (The influence of contiguous kinetic (motile) systems upon the production of esophageal speech. *Arch Ohr Nas Kehlkopfheilk, 173:*529–33.

Wepman, J.M.; MacGahan, J.A.; Richard, J.C., and Shelton, N.W. (1953): The objective measurement of progressive esophageal speech development. *J Speech Hearing Dis, 18:*247–51.

West, R.; Ansberry, M., and Carr, A. (1957): *The Rehabilitation of Speech,* 3rd rev. ed. New York, Harper and Row.

Wintersteen, L.L. (1963): Speech rehabilitation of the laryngectomized person. *Arch Phys Med Rehab, 44:*454–56.

Appendix

DIRECTORY OF SOURCES OF SUPPLY FOR ITEMS OF BENEFIT TO LARYNGECTOMEES*

Note: Neither the author nor IAL endorse or recommend any item mentioned in this list. The IAL and the author respect the ethical practices of the medical profession in every way. It is urged that no one use this directory in any way for commercial advantage. Specifications for any item should be obtained from the supplier mentioned.

TRACHEA TUBES, OBDURATORS

The surgeon recommends specific sizes for each patient. They are obtainable from local surgical supply houses. Some clubs have tubes for loan.

BIBS, AIR FILTERS (knitted, crocheted, gauze)

Local Lost Chord Clubs make these for sale to members.

IAL Office, 219 E. 42nd Street, New York, N.Y. 10017 has instructions for making bibs, nylon type.

New York Anamilo Club, 61 Irving Place, New York, N.Y. 10003 has instructions for making bibs, nylon type.

Patterns for bibs and neckwear may be obtained from an 8½ x 11-inch pamphlet prepared by "SALS," laryngectomized women. This is distributed by the IAL Office.

STOMA SCREENS AND FILTERS

Claude Crowell, 112 N. Seminole Circle, Ft. Wayne, Ind. 46807.

Kenneth Lockwood, 5035 Lily St. Place, Pinellas Park, Fla. 33565.

Martindale Electric Company, Box 617, Edgewater Branch, Cleveland, Ohio 44107.

John McClear, 61 Irving Place, New York, N.Y. 10003.

Mine Safety Appliances Company, 201 N. Braddock Ave., Pittsburgh, Pa. 15208.

Stoma Filter Button Co., 11100 Venice Boulevard, Culver City, Calif. 90230.

*Published with the permission of the IAL. Some addenda were inserted by the author.

ABA Surgical Co., P.O. Box 55, High Point, N.C. 27461.
United Surgical Co., 152 Midland Avenue, Port Chester, N.Y. 10573.
Vincent C. Hozier, 12012 Herbert Street, Los Angeles, Calif. 90066.

ASPIRATORS (heavy-duty or portable)
Local offices of the American Cancer Society in some cities may loan
aspirators to newly laryngectomized patients. Otherwise, they may
be rented from local surgical supply houses with the surgeon's recommendations.

SHOWER COLLARS
C.L. Sheldon, 462 Mt. Auburn Street, Watertown, Mass. 02172.

HOME HUMIDIFIERS
Electric type: Local appliance dealers.
Permanent type: Local plumbing firms (for installation on the heating
plant). Get specifications for degree of moisture from the surgeon.

EMERGENCY IDENTIFICATION AND WARNING
Bracelet type: Medic-Alert Foundation, 1030 Sierra Drive, Turlock,
Calif. 95380. (*Note:* Any drugstore will order a bracelet or neck
piece, printing thereon the person's medical problem and advice.)
Pocket card type: IAL Office.
Auto shield sticker: Emergency warning to police. IAL Office.
Civil Defense card: obtainable from local Civil Defense office.

MANUALS OF INSTRUCTION IN POSTLARYNGECTOMY SPEECH
Esophageal Speech, by Mary Doehler; also in French. American Cancer
Society, 138 Newbury Street, Boston, Mass. 02116.
Your New Voice, by W.F. Waldrop and M.A. Gould. American Cancer
Society, local units and state divisions.
How To Speak Again, by M. Hyman and M.S. Keller. Dr. Melvin
Hyman, Speech Department, Bowling Green State University,
Bowling Green, Ohio 43402.
Self-help for the Laryngectomee (revised), by Edmund Lauder, 6334
Dove Hill Drive, San Antonio, Tex. 78238.
Your Second Voice, by John McClear. Speech Rehabilitation Institute,
61 Irving Place, New York, N.Y. 10003.

PHONOGRAPH RECORDS FOR POSTLARYNGECTOMY SPEECH INSTRUCTION
Mrs. Paul A. Doehler, 243 Charles Street, Boston, Mass. 02114.
Dr. Melvin Hyman, Speech Department, Bowling Green State University, Bowling Green, Ohio 43402.

ARTIFICIAL LARYNGES
Aurex Corp., 315 W. Adams Street, Chicago, Ill. 60606.
Kett Engineering Co., 2444 Wilshire Boulevard, Santa Monica, Calif. 90403.
Rand Development Corp., 13600 Deise Avenue, Cleveland 44110.
Bell Telephone Co. (Apply to any local office for the electronic instrument and parts for your old pneumatic instruments.)
Rev. Y. Yamamura, Amaki Kurasiki City, Japan, for inexpensive pneumatic.
Technisch Bureau MEMACVON, P.O. Box 56, Velp (G) Holland (van Hunen Larynx).

AMPLIFIERS FOR WEAK VOICES
Brenkert & Deming, Box 47, Royal Oak, Mich. 48068.
IAL Office, 219 E. 42nd Street, New York, N.Y. 10017 for plans for making an amplifier.
A.R. Mann, 1560 W. William Street, Decatur, Ill. 62522.
Paulon Blaney Research, Inc., c/o Lions Industry for the Blind, 7810 S. Dixie, West Palm Beach, Fla. 33405.
Portable Rostrum, amplifier built in plastic frame for lectures. Uses DC and AC current. Available at radio dealers.
Power Page Megaphone No. 2. University Loudspeakers Inc., 80 S. Kenseco Place, White Plains, N.Y.

TAPE RECORDERS
Available in radio and department stores. Caution: Only high quality instruments are advised for good fidelity; get advice from speech center.

TOK-BAK, 2926 Avalon Avenue, Berkeley, Calif. 94705.
A Y-shaped, semiround plastic tube. With the Y end held before the mouth and two ends over the ears, voiced sound is carried to the ears, giving good feedback. A very useful and practical device for training persons to hear themselves.

PUBLICATIONS OF THE IAL

IAL News. Published bimonthly—free.

Directory. Published annually—includes Officers, Directors, Advisors and committees, as well as affiliated clubs, their officers, meeting dates, places and times; and facilities for speech instruction. 66 pages.

Laryngectomees' Manual. The IAL program for local chapters of the American Cancer Society. Contains instructions on basic organization and program for Lost Chord Clubs. 22 pages.

First-Aid for Laryngectomees (pamphlet). Gives special instructions for first aid to laryngectomees. For distribution to all kinds of public safety officials. Available through the local office of the American Cancer Society or the local Lost Chord Clubs (Code #3015). 10 pages.

Bibliography on Rehabilitation of Laryngectomees. Lists articles of interest to members of the medical profession and postlaryngectomy speech instructors. Revised 1967. 26 pages. *Note:* Snidecor's (1968) text contains 833 items from worldwide sources.

Helping Words (pamphlet)—illustrated. To be given to the newly laryngectomized. Gently explains what has happened, and how the patient can live a normal life in the future. For distribution by doctors and competent laryngectomees. Available through the local office of the American Cancer Society or the local Lost Chord Club (Code #4511). 22 pages.

Rehabilitating Laryngectomees (pamphlet). For use as a giveaway piece at lectures and exhibits, and for new patients. Available through the local office of the American Cancer Society (Code #4506). 10 pages.

Laryngectomees at Work (pamphlet)—illustrated. A direct appeal to employers to encourage them to employ or reemploy laryngectomees (Code #4519). 8 pages.

Speakers' Source Book for Laryngectomees. Facts, figures and tips for laryngectomized speakers. Excellent material for talks before nursing classes, service clubs and church groups.

REPRINTS

The IAL prepares printings of addresses and proceedings of annual meetings. It also duplicates or obtains reprints of timely articles that are of interest to speech pathologists and teachers of esophageal speech.

EXHIBITS

"Esophageal Speech Following Laryngectomy" (10' x 3'). This is a full-sized exhibit for professional meetings, etc.

"Esophageal Speech Following Laryngectomy" (3′ x 5′). A copy of the same exhibit as above, but can be used at smaller meetings.

OTHER PUBLICATIONS

Archives of Otolaryngology and *Archives of Environmental Health*. American Medical Association, 535 N. Dearborn Street, Chicago, Ill. 60610.

FILMS

The following films are available for medical use only. They may be obtained from the Audio-Visual Department of the American Medical Association, 535 N. Dearborn Street, Chicago. Ill. 60610.

Total Laryngectomy for Carcinoma. D.R. Weaver, M.D. 3 reels, 1,200 ft, 35 minutes, color, silent. 1948 (Code #HN-2).

Organic Disorders of the Larynx. P.H. Holinger, M.D. 1 reel, 800 ft, 22 minutes, color, silent. 1947 (Code #HN-6).

Head and Neck Cancer. Presented by Hayes Martin, M.D. A kinescope of a closed-circuit TV film. 16 mm, color, sound, 45 minutes (Code #3424).

Cancer Detection. Presented by Emerson Day, M.D. A kinescope of a closed-circuit TV film. 16 mm, color, sound, 38 minutes (Code #3440).

The following film may be obtained from the Department of Medical Communications, University of Kansas Medical Center, Kansas City, Kans. 66103. Rental fee $3.00. May also be purchased from the producer.

Alaryngeal Speech. Produced by W.M. Diedrich, Ph.D., and the Department of Medical Communications, University of Kansas Medical Center. 16 mm, 20 minutes, black and white with sound. The film demonstrates one method of teaching postlaryngeal voice.

The following films should be ordered through the local office or the state division of the American Cancer Society. It is wise to review them before showing because some are now over twenty years old and may display teaching material that is no longer used.

Rehabilitation of Laryngectomized Patient (We Speak Again). Leroy A. Schall, M.D. 1 reel, 800 ft, 22 minutes, color, sound. 1949 (Code #57).

Speech After Laryngectomy. Syracuse University—Commercial Motion Pictures, 1480 Salt Springs Road, Syracuse, N.Y. 1 reel, 800 ft, 22 minutes, color, sound. 1956 (Code #58).

The Irritating Angel. Kinescope of TV program of April 26, 1959. 16 mm, black and white, sound, 28½ minutes (Code #16).

Never Alone. The American Cancer Society. Includes scenes about laryngectomees. 16 mm (also 35 mm), black and white, 28 minutes, sound. (Also, short version, *I Ate a Peach.*)

Cry Out in Silence. Kinescope of "Alcoa Premiere" TV program of May 15, 1962. 16 mm, black and white, sound, 28 minutes.

A Second Voice. A new IAL film about total rehabilitation of the laryngectomee. 16 mm, sound, color, 14 minutes (Code #81).

To Speak Again. 8 mm cartridge, color, sound, 15 minutes, used on Fairchild projector only, in hospital room. Patient can operate it. Columbia Division, American Cancer Society, Washington, D.C.

Principles of Teaching Speech After Laryngectomy. 16 mm, sound, color, 21 minutes. Narrator: James C. Shanks. Produced by American Cancer Society.

NAME INDEX

ABA Surgical Co., 26, 224

American Cancer Society, VIII, XII, 11, 18, 27, 31, 189, 190–192, 196, 209, 225, 229

American Medical Association, VIII, 20, 26, 54, 57, 65–66, 71, 104, 195, 226, 228

American Speech and Hearing Association, 71–72

Anderson, J.O., 37, 144, 215

Anderson, V., 142, 215

Andrews, A.H. Jr., 7, 14, 68, 215

Archives of Environmental Health, VIII, 228

Archives of Otolaryngology, IX, 228

Arnold, G.E., 53, 159, 215

Asai, R., 51

Augenstein, P., 99

Aurex Corp., 55–56, 226

Baker, G.L., 40, 69, 215

Bangs, J.L., Lierle, D.M. and Strother, C.R., 61, 80–83, 215

Barney, H.L., 52, 215

Barton, J. and Hejna. R., 173, 215

Bateman, G.H., 44, 215

Bateman, G.H. and Negus, V.E., 35, 215

Bateman, G.H., Dornhorst, A. and Leathhart, G., 40, 215

Beck, J., 43, 215

Behringer, S.M., 71, 215

Bell Telephone Co., 53, 57, 226

Berg, J. van den and Moolenaar-Bijl, A.J., 46, 88, 215

Berg, J. van den, Moolenaar-Bijl, A.J. and Damste, P.H., 35, 40–41, 43–45, 47–48, 149, 215

Berlin, C.I., 35–36, 41, 44, 46, 71, 75, 88, 91, 93, 97–98, 108, 129, 149, 159, 215

Berry, M.E. and Eisonsen, J., 12, 69, 215

Billroth, (quoted by Gussenbauer), XI,

Bisi, R.H. and Conley, J.J., 84, 215

Bondarenko, E.D., 68, 215

Brenkert and Deming, 226

Brighton, G.R. and Boone, W.H., 35, 215

Brodnitz, F.S., 7, 11, 30, 43, 61, 82, 215

Bureau of Vocational Rehabilitation, 29, 31, 196, 198

Chen, L.C.Y., Samberg, H.M., and Felsenstein, B. 68, 80, 85, 216

Civil Defense Office, 225

Clark, A.F., 70, 216

Cleveland Clinic Foundation, VIII, 34

Cleveland Hearing and Speech Center, VIII

Cleveland Lost Chord Club, VIII, 16, 99

Cojazzi, L., 43, 216

Conley, J.J., Deamsti, F., and Pierce, M.K., 51, 216

Cooper, H.K., 58

Cooper, Les, 72

Corgill, D.A., 70–71, 216

Crouse, G.P., 60, 216

Crowell, C., 224

Curran, V., 70, 216

Czermak, J., XI, 216

Czermak, J. and Brucke, 53

Damste, P.H., IX, XI, 3, 4, 7, 16, 33–36, 38–41, 43–46, 48–50, 52, 63, 70, 75, 80, 82–89, 91, 103, 138, 158–159, 164, 190, 197–198, 216

Damste, P.H., Berg, J. van den and Moolenaar-Bijl, A.J., 50, 61, 84, 159, 164, 216

Darley, F.L., 7, 13, 36, 38, 40, 75, 84, 86, 216

Day, E., 228

Decroix, G.; Libersa, C. and Lattard, R., 33, 216

Detroit Anamilo Club, 18

DiCarlo, L.M., Amster, W. and Herer, G., 7, 37, 48, 60, 85, 87, 142, 144, 216

Diedrich, W.M. and Youngstrom, K., IX, XI, 3, 5–6, 13–14, 17, 20, 25, 27, 30–31, 33, 50, 52–54, 58–63, 66–68, 74, 76–77, 79–80, 82–83, 86–89, 91, 97, 103, 114–118, 138, 144, 156, 158–164, 167, 169, 182–186, 198, 208, 216

Doehler, M.E., 43, 156, 225, 226

Ehrlich, N., XI, 216

Equen, M., 61, 76, 216

Ferguson, J.D., 7, 70, 216

Finkbeiner, E. R., 91, 216

Fisher, W.R., 12, 14, 219

Fletcher, H., 38, 216

Fontaine, A. and Mitchell, J., 3, 68, 84, 216

Fortune, G.J., VIII

231

SUBJECT INDEX

A

ABC's in practice, 126

Accent, *see* Loudness

Adjustments through speech therapy, 32–33, *see also* Chap. 8

Aerophagia, injection in, 46

Age vs speech skill, *see* Speech skill

Age, worries over old, 14

Aged, teaching esophageal speech to, 92
 problems of, *see* Speech, Geriatrics

Aids to laryngectomees, auditory and visual, 31
 for injection, *see* Air-charge

Air chamber, 33, 35, 46

Air-charge, 35–46, *see also* Footnote, 11[7]
 counting numbers per, 98
 inhalation for speech, 42–43, 117, 118, 161
  different from injection, 42
  sucking, 43
  tongue action during, 36
 inhalers, incidence of users, 39
 injection, 38–46
  aids, food, liquids for, 159
  air-splitting by /s/, 41, 49
  bumping of tongue during, 44
  compression by, 107
  glossal, glossopharyngeal press, 50
   different from swallow, 44
  incidence of users, 39
  initiating, with liquids, 116–117
  intraphrase type of, 185
  longer words, phrase per, 49
  nature of, 42
  new air supply, 35
  plosive sounds in, 38
  pumping, piston, action in, 40, 44, 50, 103
  scars, tightness hindrance to, 164
  sequence of injection-plosion, 41
  sniff as aid to, 118
  testing speed of, 96
  tongue-lock for, 41
  whistle technique to initiate, 156
 swallowing, 43–44, *see also* Injection
  automatized for speech, 45, 48
   see also Air in fast, out fast

delay of air intake by, 45
first stage of, 41, 114
injection as minimal, 115
liquids for speeding, 46
modified, 43–44
muscle patterns in injection and, 45–46
postlaryngectomy speed of, 45–46
syllables per, 95, 98, 136

Air expulsion, 35–36, 44, 46–48, 119
 see also Footnote, 35
 abdominal support during, 48, 119
 aided by pressure in thoracic cavity, 47
 contributors to, 35
 esophageal pressure during, 47
 expiration during, 119
 /s/ as aid to, 41

Alcoholism, 30, 32, *see also* Physical factors

Air in fast, out fast, 46

American Cancer Society, XII, *see also* Name Index
 supporting IAL, 189–192

Amplification
 by amplifier, 63–64
 by TOK-BAK, 101, 124, 161, 226
 for weak voices, 64–65, 226

Anatomical changes from laryngectomy, 33–34
 see also Footnote, 33

Anxiety, *see* Psychological problems

Arthur the Rat, 137

Articulation
 dual roles of tongue during, 38
 lack of pulmonary support during, 37
 least intelligible esophageal speech sounds, 37
 modification of, during esophageal speech, 38
 pattern differences of, 58–60
 plosive contribution to, 38
 soft palate function during, 37
 vowel stability during, 37

Artificial larynx
 advantages, disadvantages, 14, 60
 bases of speech with, 58–60
 demonstrated, 99, 167
 emphasis with, 179
 hand assembled type, 56
 history, 52–53, *see also* Footnote, 53
 manufacturers, *see* Appendix